THE BIG BEAUTY BOOK

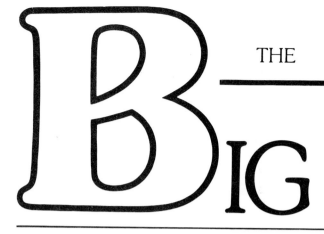

THE

BIG
BEAUTY
BOOK

GLAMOUR FOR THE
FULLER-FIGURE
WOMAN

by Ann Harper and Glenn Lewis

SIDGWICK & JACKSON/LONDON

PHOTO CREDITS

p. 23: Robert Barclay Studios for Lady Anabelle
Lingerie; pp. 25-27, 49, 51, 52, 55, 60, 62, 65-68: Bill
Morris (hair and makeup, Jimmy Weis); p. 40: Jeff
Sleppin (hair and makeup, Rick Caldwell); p. 46: Roger
Prigent; pp. 76, 106, 108, 110-112, 114, 146: Mark
Bugzester; p. 79, top left: Umberto Bertoli for Kayser
Roth; p. 79, bottom left: William Connors for "Young
Stuff"; p. 79, right: Nancy LeVine for *Harper's Bazaar*
(hair and makeup, Gary Gale); p. 87: Mark Bugzester
(hair and makeup, Rick Caldwell); pp. 157, 159, 161:
Christopher Micaud (hair and makeup, Jimmy Weis); pp.
166, 168; 170-179: Christopher Micaud.

FASHION CREDITS

chapters 3 and 10: Unitard courtesy of Danskin; chapter
7: dresses and striped top and skirt courtesy of Ashanti, a
boutique in New York; skirt suits courtesy of The Classic
Woman by Evan Picone; pants suit separates courtesy of
E.F. Benson; chapter 9: swimsuit courtesy of Robby Len
Swimwear.

ILLUSTRATIONS BY E. OVERALL

First published in Great Britain in 1984
by Sidgwick & Jackson Limited.
First softcover edition 1985

Originally published in the United States
of America in 1983 by Holt, Rinehart and Winston.

Reprinted January 1985

ISBN: 0-283-99129-1 (hardcover)
ISBN: 0-283-99248-4 (softcover)

Printed in Great Britain by
R. J. Acford, Industrial Estate, Chichester, Sussex
for Sidgwick & Jackson Limited
1 Tavistock Chambers, Bloomsbury Way
London WC1A 2SG

CONTENTS

FOREWORD

A whole division of Ford Models, Inc. was built around Ann Harper, who became our first fuller-figure model in August, 1978.

She was much better received than the other "pioneers" in this field. The image she presented seemed more glamorous and contemporary. Her photos combined an exquisite face with a youthful, well-proportioned body. Consumers found her to be refreshingly confident.

Manufacturers were also taken with Ann's bold new look and began to see the big-woman market in a different light. What started as scattered ads in the back pages of trade journals exploded into expansive national campaigns. Ann introduced a full-size line of designer jeans in a series of sexy television commercials. In addition, she launched stylish improvements in size-16-and-over hosiery, sportswear, leotards, and swimsuits for several other high-visibility accounts.

By 1980, Ann was firmly established as the most recognizable model for a rapidly growing industry, and millions of glamour-hungry women were spending billions of dollars a year on a new array of smartly designed clothes. Ann emerged as a symbol of where this fuller-figure revolution was heading. She traveled around the country for a number of key manufacturers staging impromptu fashion shows at major department stores. Almost all the models for these informal presentations were local women drafted from the audiences.

Ann would take the novice models under her wing for on-the-spot makeup tips, accessory pointers, and hairstyling adjustments. There would even be some quick coaching in the art of walking and carrying themselves like professionals. As Ann moderated, the made-over ladies paraded one by one in front of friends, relatives, and peers. Many of them were feeling truly glamorous for the first time in their lives.

The real highlight of these shows, however, was always the lively question-and-answer sessions. Here the women had a chance to ask *anything and everything* relating to being big, healthy, or beautiful. Ann invariably created a marvelous, loose rapport with her audiences. *Without* lecturing, she replied in reassuring tones that provided sound guidance.

The overriding philosophy of Ann's talks

was that women should work with their size—not run away from it. She must have hit a responsive chord, for we were constantly receiving highly complimentary mail at the agency about Ann's advice. Many of the women wanted to know if we had Ann Harper glamour booklets. Did Ann send out a newsletter filled with hints from her fashion shows?

After a while, it got quite disconcerting to have to repeatedly say no. That's when I joined the chorus of voices urging Ann to collect her fuller-figure wisdom in one definitive volume. She finally heeded our call by contacting writer Glenn Lewis. The wonderful results of their collaboration fill the pages of *The Big Beauty Book*.

All of Ann Harper's tricks of the trade are laid out in a chronological program. Much of what's written is so logical, you will wonder why you didn't think of it yourself. Other parts are so clever, you will be amazed at her ingenuity. In the end, you will have a fresh lease on life as a more beautiful fuller-figure woman.

Eileen Ford

ACKNOWLEDGMENTS

It takes more people to turn out a worthwhile book than readily meets a reader's eye. *The Big Beauty Book* is no exception. Quite a few people made valuable contributions to the project. We, the authors, don't want the efforts of our friends and colleagues to be overlooked.

First, we wish to give our *special* thanks to some key contributors:

To Claudia Black of Ford Models, Inc., for introducing us to each other.

To Denis Holler who helped put the whole project together and got it well on its way.

To our superb, patient editor, Bobbi Mark; and to our diligent agent, Jay Acton.

To Francine Fialkoff for editing, listening, researching, and always caring.

To Jimmy Weis, who shared a wealth of makeup knowledge. To Kim Lepine and Louis Licari for sharing their hairstyling and coloring knowledge, care, and attention.

To Denise Keegan for typing, proofing, and photocopying beyond the call of duty.

To Lee Overall for her painstaking illustrations.

Others deserving our appreciation are Dorothy Pollack of Formfit Rogers; Nat Drutman of Evan Picone; John Lo Morro of Evan Picone; Robert Barclay Studios; Joy Farenden of Lady Annabelle; Jill Levener, editor-in-chief of Butterick Patterns; Geraldine Onorato of *Harper's Bazaar;* Joyce Knoller of Danskin; Gurney's Inn, Montauk, New York; photographer Mark Bugzester; photographer Bill Morris; photographer Christopher Micaud; Dr. Stephen J. Manocchio; Dr. James P. B. Lynch; Arlene Redmond; chief nutritionist for the Obesity Clinic at St. Luke's Hospital; Martin Wallace, vitamin and nutrition expert; Steve Austin; Pat Williams of Ashanti; Ronnie Levine of Robby Len Swimwear; all the great people at Stout Sportswear Group; Max and Sarah; and most of all Bunny!

We also want to recognize the strong support of our families and close friends. Their understanding made the months of continual work much more tolerable.

April 25, 1982

Ann Harper
Glenn Lewis

PART ONE

SIZING YOURSELF DOWN

CHAPTER ONE

SOULMATES

Glamour is an alluring personal style that fascinates the people who come in contact with it. Despite what you've heard all your life, it doesn't come in only petite sizes or super-thin packages. Any large woman can be truly glamorous if she learns to make the most of her looks and goes after beauty with an "I won't be denied" attitude.

As a model, my secret weapon is to meet the chic "skinnies" head on with no apologies. Recently, in fact, I was one of three fuller-figure models mixed in with twenty perfect size-6 women in a fashion show at a New York City department store. When I arrived backstage the sight of all those sleek torsos made my palms a bit moist with anxiety. But let's face it, there's no place for me to hide in

a room where almost everybody is sixty pounds lighter and ten dress sizes smaller. So, I took a deep breath before setting out to transform myself into a strikingly *unavoidable* creature.

By overstating my positive features, size suddenly became an asset. Makeup dramatically accentuated the flash of my hazel eyes, the fullness of my lips, and the broadness of my cheekbones. Elaborate accessories, too overpowering for a slightly built girl, added color and dazzle to a pale blue outfit. Even my bustline and hips became more sensuous by adding a wide, supposedly taboo belt to a linen suit with a kick-pleat skirt. Believe me, my good points weren't going to be washed away in the harsh runway lights.

The first group of models lined up behind the curtain in order of appearance. Five skinnies in various red, white, or blue spring creations with me as, pardon the pun, the anchor. While we psyched ourselves up for the show, several hands fluttered around us tugging here, flattening there, straightening, fixing, fussing. One girl in front of me wore a suit identical to mine, except for the color. She glared at me for a moment. Imagine, a size 16 nervy enough to wear the same outfit as she! And she became downright angry when a stylish wide-brimmed hat was plucked from her head and given to me.

A moment later a few hundred people applauded, and Frank "Old Blue Eyes" Sinatra crooned "New York, New York," as we gathered at center stage to pose a scene. My dressalike regally crooked a wrist as if checking her watch, two models froze back to back with arms folded, another pair of skinnies leaned motionless shoulder against shoulder, and I put both hands to my hips in mock impatience. Suddenly, the music shifted to a pulsating rock rhythm, which set the girls into action one after the other down the runway. The audience greeted their graceful spins and turns with silence, a hush of awe. These flawless nymphs, without the fleshy meat of reality, came across as a distant fantasy in the glow of the footlights.

Finally, it was my turn. I heard Donna Summer's sexy voice grinding out "Bad Girls." My adrenaline rose to the music and put me in a confident, naughty mood. I gave a knowing smile, paused, tugged suggestively at the brim of my hat. The crowd behind the lights cheered, clapped, even answered with a few shrill whistles. During my strut and whirls down the runway the noise built. I could begin to make out some of the shouts.

"All right!" yelled an athletically husky blond about my age. "Show them how sexy we are."

"Hey, I could wear that suit," said a noticeably ample woman in the second row, nudging her equally excited husband. "Does that come in purple?"

"What size are *you*, honey? I'm not much bigger than you, I bet." A woman to my right stood and seemed to examine her body as if seeing it for the first time.

The one comment from the audience that affected me the most came in a stage whisper. "You're big! You mean I could be a fashion model?" I glanced down at my feet to see a heavy, dumbfounded teenager leaning over the edge of the runway. "Na-a-ah, I'm still too fat," she decided.

Too fat! How many girls like my doubting admirer have allowed those words to crush their aspirations? I remember insecure days when my craving for the limelight was frustrated by being *too fat*. My father owned the Village Barn, a Manhattan nightclub, where cabaret acts drew wildly enthusiastic responses. From adolescence on, all I ever wanted out of life was to sing to an ovation.

Everybody told me that my voice was good enough and that I had definite stage presence. But it's hard to play the heroine in a high school musical when you dwarf your leading man. Like most of us big women, I was a painfully huge, prematurely developed kid. Standing 5 feet 8 inches, and weighing 157 pounds at twelve years old was awkward. Add a snug-fitting 36-B bra and I began to feel something like Mae West in the land of the Munchkins.

When I was a child, my mother made the age-old mistake of using food as a reward. By the time my body started to blossom, food became a form of protective camouflage. Oh, the innocent stupidity of trying to cover up our ripening breasts and broadening hips under a layer of fat. The choice, to my way of thinking, boiled down to being either a woman in the world of gawking, grabby teenagers or just another overweight girl in the group. I ran from the burdens of womanhood and hid in the cookie jar.

In the following years, my visions of stardom dominated frequent daydreams, but more and more food became my way of handling the real-life problems. Come on ladies, you all know the patterns. Meet a few strangers at a friend's house and the next thing you know a piece of cake is your excuse for not having to say something clever. Squabble with a loved one and soak up the acidity in your stomach with a quart or two of ice cream. Lose the affection of the man you yearn for and compensate with a warm, rich five-course hug.

A-a-ah, the food caresses your aching heart delicately from the inside. It fills you with a satisfying desire. Who really loves ya, darling? Why, loyal, dependable, never-going-to-leave-you F-O-O-D, of course.

The emotional bond between the compulsive eater and her daily fix of assorted goodies is not a smooth, predictable relationship. My comforting romances with overeating usually turn into a startlingly vicious, roller-coaster kind of affair. Many of you might know it better as the old "yo-yo syndrome": eat tons, lose weight fast, eat up again. In a cycle similar to the uncontrolable highs and lows of heroin, it jerks your ego abruptly from one extreme to the other. The physical effects can be draining and sometimes almost as harmful as a bad drug habit.

Yo-yoing begins by suppressing all sorts of day-to-day hurts with a plunge into gluttony. I shovel down cake, candy, any food, in gulps that I consume without actually tasting. The idea of falling back into the binging doldrums, the same old patterns, brings on an unshakable guilt. In an effort to turn things around and overcome the guilt, I shift to a plan of self-denial. I try to balance the sinful overeating with a body-torturing crash diet. Naturally, I reward myself for losing weight with a fresh bouquet of calories. Once again, five pounds heavier than when I started, my appetite swells ready to devour a new hurt.

Somehow, we compulsive eaters manage to convince ourselves that the present binge is well under control. We constantly mouth the same little lies all other addicts use:

"I can end this pig-out whenever I want." Sound familiar?

"One more day of this before I drop my fork and go outside." Didn't you say that yesterday?

"It's a cloudy, dreary weekend anyway." Open the blinds and see the sun, my dear.

"I swear, no matter what happens, this is the last time I go hog wild!" Sure, you're the boss.

My personal illusions of self-control were eventually shattered by one bottomless, spirit-engulfing binge. After I graduated from college, the years of wishing for singing stardom were over. My make-believe crutch was taken away, and the fear of failure really crippled me. Fall auditions promised to be a series of humiliating scenes that would leave me without any alternatives. I decided as early as May that nobody would hire an unknown singer who was twice the size of any girl in the chorus line.

That summer our family had a house at the shore. In preparation for the death of my career, I began to bury myself as soon as we arrived. The world of thin people was out there waiting to embarrass me. Well, they would have to dig through walls of brick, gloom, and fat to find me. I just closed myself in for the next three months with my TV, nagging self-doubts, and a full refrigerator.

On hot, sunny days my older sister Ruth and our friends socialized in the sand with guys from the area, swam, and worked on developing bronzy tans. They badgered me to join them, but for a suffocating starlet the beach seemed a thousand miles away. What little energy I expended was reserved for tricky eating maneuvers. I played the very same food games that hell-bent noshers have been involved in since Betty Crocker was a short-cake. Sweets vanishing, reappearing, and mysteriously gone again. Nobody could blame me, I figured. None of them ever caught me in the act.

The family was accustomed to waking up by mid-morning, so I rolled out of bed at the crack of dawn—to jam in a platter of thickly buttered pancakes slathered with syrup. My timing was right on the money. Dish, skillet, and silverware were dried and put away seconds before the rest of the clan sat down to breakfast. Yawning widely, I made a show of being the last one to the table. I even let everybody else fill their plates before taking my fair share.

Once I was left alone in the house my deceptions took a grander scale. For instance, I often used the celebrated "piece o' pie switch-eroo." The name might be unfamiliar, but I'm quite sure a few of you will recognize the ploy. It worked well enough that summer to account all by itself for ten new pounds.

Invariably, a day-old chocolate cream pie was left very prominently displayed in the refrigerator. Every member of the family was keenly aware that only a single wedge had been eaten. In fact, they each reminded me of it before leaving for the beach. Oh, I burned for that pie! All the fat cells in my body reached out to it.

Ten seconds after the door slammed, I was breathlessly picking at the gooey confection. One forkful rhythmically followed another. Soon, the tin was empty and panic took over. In a rare burst of vitality, I raced three blocks to buy a fresh pie. Back home, I realized that my heist wasn't yet fully concealed. You guessed it. I downed a piece that perfectly matched the section missing from the original chocolate cream pie. Outrageous—a whole fabulous pie bites the dust, and I appear to be gutsy Ms. Willpower.

The pretending stopped early in August. By Labor Day weekend I was too depressed and bloated to hide anything. My weight had climbed in three months from 175 pounds to a sloppy 210. Clothes bulged at the seams. Muscle tone was totally shot. Skulking around the house in a daze, I gorged myself openly and was too miserable even to bother combing my hair.

My sister had been quietly sympathetic during most of the binge, but took the standard "let it run its course" approach to the problem. After all, she knew exactly what I was going through. Ruth had experienced numbing, food-crazed months of her own. Barely an inch over five feet tall, she remembered weighing as much as 160 pounds and still kept size-16½ dresses stashed in the rear of her closet—brakes to prevent backsliding, she called them. Now, Ruth had been maintaining a trim, lighter body for two straight years and seemed so level, so genuinely happy.

Ruth sat me down to talk out my anxieties when it became obvious that the upswing in the yo-yo syndrome was way overdue. First, she reminisced about her own fat, desperate days. The fears she referred to were my own fears. It was as if she were mouthing all the frightening thoughts locked inside me. I wanted to agree with everything she said. Finally, I found myself interrupting her with an unchecked flood of words. My obsessive anticipation of rejection was no longer a terrifying secret. It was being shared, and the release made me feel sort of giddy. We were closer than sisters at that moment. Ruth had become my soul mate.

Together we took stock of who I *really* was. What were the most practical solutions to my problems? Ruth began to put things in focus by helping me to list my positive physical features. She started me off by noting that a 5-foot-9½-inch woman was tall enough to carry some extra weight. Great! One good point to my credit. And there's . . . uhhhh . . . ummmm . . . . I was stumped.

Again, Ruth to the rescue. She told me how lucky I was to have pounds that were evenly distributed. I guess that was true. My body was just as overburdened on top as it was in the middle or down below. And despite rampant fat cells elsewhere, my legs were quite shapely. Okay, that makes three indisputable pluses. Yeah, and the plumpness of my cheeks couldn't totally hide those hazel eyes, regular nose, and white, pearly teeth. Also, my hair was healthy, my chin was strong, my posture was correct, my . . . .

Hey, not bad! Sure I knew I was still pudgy, but I didn't visualize myself as so ugly after that. Those were the credentials of a beautiful woman. Maybe a disguised beautiful woman. Maybe even a distorted beautiful woman. It frankly didn't matter. The possibilities were making me overanxious for results. "I definitely could be a knockout," I blurted out. "If there were only a way to shed seventy, eighty, or ninety pounds in a hurry."

Ruth recognized all the signs. DANGER! Here comes another stomach-rattling crash diet. Once again, it was time to get me in check. She tried to convince me that a gradual diet was healthier and a lot less frustrating. Losing it all at once was an impossible task. Even if you dropped a few pounds, it was always counted as a dismal failure.

"No, I have to lose ninety pounds now," I insisted. "Can you imagine how incredible

I'd look in a size-ten dress? That's when I would be beautiful."

Ruth then told me, in ultradirect terms, the hard-and-true limitations of my body. Broad shoulders, large thighs, wide hips, and a sluggish metabolism don't fit into a pixie figure. My parts were clearly too buxom to add up to a 120-pound gal. The message was there in plain language. *There isn't any size-10 pot of gold at the end of my rainbow.*

Wait a minute! I was stunned. It's not easy giving up every diet book's version of the "skinny you." Good heavens, I was forsaking the Pepsi generation, deserting Jack LaLanne's streamlined army, denying the gospel according to *Vogue*. It was social blasphemy. Yet, deep down I knew Ruth was right. I was an unfit size 22 who would be old and decrepit before ever being thin.

Fortunately, my disappointment didn't last very long. Our chats suggested another appealing, vastly more plausible objective. By studying my structural blessings and pitfalls, I realized that I could be a gorgeous, solid size 16 without too much work. It was a long-range plan that I could tackle in three-week segments. And it was the first shape-up goal I fully expected to accomplish.

Ruth wanted me to savor success as soon as possible. So she asked me to lose just five pounds in the first three weeks. As added incentive, a nonfood reward was dangled in front of me. Less than a month of clean living, losing those five pounds, and picking up a silk scarf or pendulous earrings as a bonus. It was just the opposite of my vicious cycles. Instead of a depression following an

unhealthy binge, I was getting a gift to make me feel good because I bothered to make myself look better.

My sister introduced me to the concept of quality calories. I didn't have to eat less food or even more boring meals. I simply tried to eat things that provided the most nutrition and enjoyment for the calories being consumed. A huge array of appetizing dishes were on the menu without the side orders of guilt. Granted, I had to monitor what I ate to some extent, but at least now I didn't have to hide what I was eating.

How wonderful I thought it would be to take off those five pounds and not feel defeated because size 10 was nowhere in sight. Actually, in the initial three weeks I went plummeting from 210 pounds down to 200. I know, you're probably thinking big deal—it was mostly water loss. Well, right you are, except in this instance those pounds stayed lost, and I continued to peel off the typically more stubborn fat.

In five months I was painlessly scaling the 180-pound plateau. Ruth showered me with daily comments of encouragement in her two-minute pep-rally phone calls. She sent funny "go get 'em" cards. When we passed store windows Ruth pointed out smaller dresses by saying, "Next month you'll be wearing that." It worked like a charm.

I was not *only* losing weight, I just naturally became more active, which in turn made my body firmer. The muscle-to-fat ratio in my body shifted. My social life gradually picked up, too. Listen, I wanted as many people as possible to see the new me. Why not? There seemed to be a new me in the mirror every single time I looked.

After seven months, my weight was below 170 pounds. Musical auditions were now a normal part of my schedule. Admittedly, Broadway wasn't clamoring at my feet, but I wasn't wasting away in the wings, either. It was at one of those "cattle call" auditions, an open tryout for anybody smart enough to find the theater, that my modeling career accidentally started. The stage manager persuaded me to go see an agent about modeling. I still thought that I was much too heavy, however, my revitalized vanity was whispering maybe. Bingo! Two weeks later I was offered $180 an hour to do a half-clad, queen-sized pantyhose package.

At the end of the eighth month, I reached my goal. My enlightened routine had given birth to a 165-pound happy woman. The clothes in my closet were 99 percent different from what had been hanging there during my binge days. Now, boldly cut-out size 16s in a multitude of festive pastels took up most of the racks. They were a symbol of the glorious new Ann Harper I vowed to maintain. Yet, like my soulmate, I kept a couple of oversized frocks squirreled away as reminders of another me.

Ruth's sisterly shove in the right direction brightened my whole existence. She recognized my problems, anticipated my anxieties, and cared enough to share her insights. Well, I want to do the same thing for every fuller-figure woman. I believe we're all sisters to a certain degree. No, I'm not suggesting that each size-16 and over has a similar body, or intellect, or even needs the same amount of help. However, we are closely bound by a wealth of common experiences, obstacles, and concerns.

Maybe, it's more accurate to say that we're all soul mates. Our spirits are linked by a mutual desire for glamour, health, and happiness in a society that puts stout women at a horrendous disadvantage. My years in modeling have provided me with a knack for making the most of my looks as well as access to those experts who earn a living maximizing the beauty of others. What can be more natural than letting my soul mates benefit from my good fortune?

The pages that follow will present my organized, step-by-step program for comfortably becoming the most glamorous woman you can. Throughout the book a clear-cut, pragmatic philosophy is set forth. You are asked to consistently take a positive, but honest look at yourself, to appreciate the merits and potential of your finer points. Yes, you'd be surprised at how many attributes you have. Likewise, I also expect you to own up to valid trouble spots. Don't fret! My remedies are all quite safe, often enjoyable, and tend to be very effective.

One much-too-easy piece of advice you won't get here is the "fat is fantastic" doctrine. Suddenly, it has become fashionable to tell women that excessive fat is okay. Living out of shape is marvelous. Just eat, drink, and be merry! "Put on a happy face," they say, "and you'll be beautiful." Ridiculous! Blind pats on the back will hurt terribly in the long run. They give a crippling, false sense of well-being.

I don't hesitate to say "Fat is ugly!" There is nothing aesthetically pleasing about loose, unmolded rolls of fat. We all know that's true. Why kid ourselves? But I'm quick to add, without equivocation, "Big, firm, and healthy is sensually appealing."

This book tells you to stop waiting around for the miraculous size-10 body that never comes. I want to slowly transform the unkempt, jelly-bellied size 22 into a more taut, attractive size 20. Then I want to push her on to visions of a dazzling, well-proportioned 18 dress size. By the way, women busy battling against the size-16 bulge can benefit from the same program. In fact, I might just ease them right down to a compact size 14 and out of the fuller-figure category altogether.

As preparation for the Big Beauty treatment, you will first have to establish a reassuring, workable self-image. The next chapter tries to show you how to accomplish that. It helps you cope with some common attitude problems and makes you more aware of subliminal fears that get in the way of being a complete person. Chapter 3, "Balancing Your Body," then takes a comprehensive survey of your anatomy. You'll begin to think as a definite body type with a carefully directed eye toward balance and proportion.

The rest of the book is set up like a timetable for your personal improvement. Part II provides breathtaking results in a jiffy. There, I give you a lifetime supply of *instant*

glamour tips to make you look prettier and feel more desirable immediately. My team of professionals pitch in with numerous hairstyles, makeup secrets, fashion hints, and facial routines designed for your particular specifications. You'll get just the ego boost required to pounce into the section on "Figuring the New You—Soon."

In three-week intervals you go after easy, reachable goals guaranteed to perceptively shape up your body. An enjoyable but rational food plan will allow you to take off five to ten pounds. Soft-core sports and socializing will tone lax muscles. Posture pointers will straighten you up.

"Beyond the New You—Later" is my graduate course for overachievers. The miniprogram is extended to include more demanding regimens that can translate into a year-in and year-out approach to life. I start by giving the easiest ways to maintain the new you. Then, modified recipes, vitamin supplements, and nutritional information are used to bolster your already healthy diet. To test and tighten you further, sports workouts become more rigorous. And finally, I show you how sexy and confident a fuller-figure beauty like you can be.

Whoa! Perhaps, we're getting a little ahead of ourselves. Let's go back to our first order of business—about the way you think of yourself.

CHAPTER TWO

WHO DO YOU

THINK YOU ARE?

Before we get a fix on your self-image, let me tell you about a friend of mine. Vicki is a 5-foot 6-inch 190-pounder who thinks of herself as a beautiful floating head. Don't laugh! She is just another large woman subconsciously rejecting her body. You'd be surprised how many of us do it—but usually to some lesser degree.

Vicki wakes up in the morning to her neck-up reflection in the bathroom mirror. She leans over the sink to study the fine features and baby-soft skin. Meticulously, using far too much makeup, she draws and colors in every detail. Her face shimmers iridescently over an unseen torso—like a full moon in a night sky. Light auburn hair, combed into tight curls, outlines the lunar effect.

Vicki always dresses quickly. The idea is to zip her body under a dark, drab outfit. Sort of the old "out of sight, out of mind" philosophy. Maybe, it's more the belief that "what you can't see won't hurt you." Anyhow, both clichés don't quite work for her. The body she's trying to take out of the picture winds up being difficult to avoid. Her clothes seem to be in a continuous tug-of-war with a stranger. If I put my hands over her eyes, Vicki couldn't tell me one thing about what she was wearing. She's in too much of a hurry to care.

During her working day Vicki sits behind a high reception desk. Her face is intelligently alive from the second she comes in. Animated smiles, smirks, winks, and glib talk charm the horde of people passing through her area. However, Vicki's personality never seems to reach below her chin. She often appears to be totally out of communication with herself. Vicki's arms tend to hang limply; her movements are all graceless and out of sync. And the playful sensuality in her facial expressions has nothing whatsoever to do with an absolutely passive body.

Vicki defensively defines glamour as being "Just another pretty face." But when I made her list her strong points and beauty shortcomings, she mostly jotted down complaints about her body. Oh, she hated the shape of her breasts, her rear was too big, her legs were too short, and her thighs looked like "saddlebags." Standard large-woman complaints.

What she didn't know was that these were also standard size-8 complaints. Ask an attractive size-8 woman to list her pluses and minuses and she'd sound exactly like a size-28 Weight Watchers dropout. My experiences have shown me that almost no woman, no matter what size and shape she's in, is ever satisfied with the way her body looks. Fuller-figure women just take it for granted that it's easier to cope with the anxieties of a smaller frame. But size-8 sisters agonize over their breasts, find their bottoms too sprawling, and cross their legs to hide their flabby thighs—just like the rest of us.

Overall glamour for the heavy, thin, short, or tall must begin by accepting your body. Learn to live within your present physique, not in spite of it. Get in touch with the size you are—be it a 12, 16, or 26—rather than run away from the shapeless form you *think* you are. Become familiar with the strengths of your body and its potential for improvement. How you got to this size isn't important now. Concentrate on being open, active, and at ease with your figure.

Over the years I've exhibited just about every poor attitude imaginable toward my body. The craziness I created for myself was amazing. I'm sure most of you are plagued by only a fraction of the same negative notions. Yet, they won't be corrected until you're able to identify them first. But be aware that we often act out our hostile feelings in deceptive or subtle ways.

Here is a quiz that includes eight of the most common self-defeating attitudes. I hope that I've been able to conquer them all. Find the ones that apply to you. Try to use my answers as a shortcut to your own solutions. These questions aren't supposed to make you feel bad. Just the opposite. Each one should make you aware of what a good, happy person you can be—if you take the time to set yourself right. A positive ego is a giant step toward becoming a vibrant Big Beauty.

Pencils ready? Eyes open and turned inward? Okay, begin!

1. Do you wear your raincoat even when the sun shines?

Sound crazy? I used to do it. It could be mid-July, ninety-five degrees, clear blue skies, and I'd be wearing an open trench coat. I wasn't comfortable with the way I looked. So I brainwashed myself into believing that a curtain of cloth would cover my folds, rolls, and general heft. Meanwhile, people gawked curiously at the perspiration dripping down my neck, under my arms, everywhere.

When I dressed this way I assumed I was alone. Poor me, the only person around who was obviously out of the mainstream. The only woman on the block with a figure overload. I was so self-conscious that I never bothered to gauge the bodies passing me on the street. What a shock I got when I finally opened my eyes to the scene around me. I was anything but alone.

After all, many of you were out there looking, acting, and even dressing just like me. Cloak-and-dagger raincoats aren't your style, you say? Fine! But I bet there are times when you sneak under the old A-line tent dress, baggy tunic, or long unbelted overblouse. They all say the same thing: "Look at me! I don't like myself." The really hideous outfits sob, "Aren't I a miserable outsider with a lot of problems. I don't deserve to wear fashionable dresses because I can't lose weight."

Why don't we all stop crying and hiding? We don't have to worry about qualifying for the mainstream. The size-16-and-over set is the closest thing to a mainstream this society has. Very few women don't have a little too much here or an excess there. For your information, government surveys and fashion-industry estimates claim that well over 30 million fuller-figure women are living in the United States. Or, approximately one out of every three women in the country is one of us.

The numbers suggest that we're the real force in the world of women. Why should we feel intimidated around size 8s? Let the string-beans worry about being substantial enough. Some of them actually do, you know. Skin-nies are the ones who cram padding in their clothing and have breast implants and silicone injections to round things out. I know one so-called fuller-figure model (really an ambitious size 14) who earns her daily bread by stuffing her bodysuit with disposable baby diapers. *She* doesn't wear raincoats in the summer. You shouldn't either.

Dress up, don't cover up. *You must start to think of yourself as a regular size.* Work with your body to make it look naturally feminine. Wear clothes that allow you to blend in with the kind of women you admire. Give yourself the same fashion alternatives that a size 8 enjoys. Viva freedom of choice! Think, act, dress, and look like the regular mainstream person you are. Please, don't create a gap between you and the best your world has to offer.

Raincoats then are for cool spring showers and dirty old men in X-rated movie theaters. Smart fuller-figure women dress to fit the occasion, their mood, and the weather. Balmy sunshine calls for light, slightly revealing, casual clothes. In other words, take a sane approach to dressing.

2. Are you in the habit of buying dresses for a smaller woman?

No, I don't mean clothes shopping for a petite sister or a slender cousin. I'm talking about purchasing smaller-sized outfits for the skinnier woman you think you should be. It goes back to a "wishing makes it so" philosophy of life. Many of you believe all you have to do is wriggle into a size-18 frock and you're no longer a size 22. More mad, self-defeating fairy tales.

Once upon a time, I also bought things a size or two smaller than my body. Other people must have seen me as a parody of the old fat-lady gag. It's the one where a huge woman walks into a dress shop and sees a tiny customer taking off a revealing evening gown. "I'll take that gown," she tells the saleswoman. "Let me see if we have it in your size," the store employee replies. "Don't bother," says the bountiful woman, "I'll wear *that* gown out."

The image that punch line evokes is really anything but funny. There's only one thing sadder than trying on garment after garment of a size much too small for you. That's buying those dresses and wearing them in public. Skirts are forever riding up. Seams cut into your underarms or split below your shoulders. Tight sleeves turn fingertips blue by cutting off the circulation in your wrists. Underwear binds, twists, rubs, and pinches because of the extra pressure. And every pound of fat on your frame is accentuated against the skintight material.

Maybe you, too, have convinced yourself that if you buy smaller dresses people will think you're a smaller size. Well, you're only fooling yourself. Nobody peeks at the label to see what size clothes you're wearing. So, why be so hung-up on mere numbers? Stop thinking of the number in your dress as a scoring system for self-worth. All that kind of thinking adds up to is new barriers between your body and the mind that has to accept it. If the darn numbers bother you so much, I suggest you take a pen and change them. Size 14 equals 1, size 16 equals 2, size

18 equals 3, and so on. Now you can flash numbers with the pipsqueaks.

Work constructively with your real size. Stop taking lunging swings at distorted shadows of a body that doesn't exist. Wearing a smaller size only makes it obvious how far from being thin you are. By wearing ample, well-fitting outfits you feel more comfortable yourself and look better to others. Today, the larger sizes also come in more appealing styles and greater variety. Start to know who you are in the fashion scene, what clothes give you real confidence, and what you can actually get away with.

You can get in the habit of buying clothes for a smaller woman soon. Just do one of two things. Either lose a little weight and tighten up the body you now have, or begin to think so positively about your current size that you give a trimmer, more compact appearance. Better still, do both!

3. Are you the big loser in an endless string of no-win diets?

When I or anybody else mentions "lose weight" you automatically think DIET! Shhh, don't go spreading this around, but I have a secret about diets. You can't win in any of the thousands of fad diets. Don't take it personally. In the long run nobody wins on the diet circuit.

I have an enormous library of diet books. My shelves literally runneth over. In the past fifteen years I've done them all. I've drowned myself with glass after glass of water, eaten only vegetables, eaten only protein, almost flown over the moon on speed, and shot myself full of HCG (Hydro Corionic Gonadatrophin, which is a hormone extracted from the urine of pregnant women). Some of the other diets are too depressing to even discuss. Anyway, they all worked. Every last one of them. But only for a little while.

A victory in sports takes only a short time to accomplish. However, the winner of a particular game or specific championship has that triumph to their credit forever. Diets may last a week, two weeks, or possibly a month. Usually you lose a few pounds, but a month later you're back to your original weight. Those are no-win diets. Where is the permanent triumph or victorious new figure?

These diets just are not designed to last. None of them even remotely considers the basic eating needs fuller-figure women have developed in the course of their lives. We all, especially me, *love* food! Or we believe we do. We see food as a source of enjoyment. Sure, we can force ourselves to give up almost anything for days or even weeks. But to totally give up the pleasures of diversified eating for years? Pure foolishness!

The road to daily happiness isn't deprivation. Stop making diets your form of public penance for being heavy. How many of you can walk down a street and feel comfortable about eating an ice cream cone? Very few, I'll wager. You feel people are staring at you and commenting on your size, maybe thinking to themselves, "She wouldn't be that size if she gave up that cone." Well, most likely they're not thinking that. And giving up the ice cream is not the answer to all your weight problems.

There isn't any reason why you can't eat almost any kind of food you desire. In theory, you can have a portion of your cake or ice cream and lose pounds too. The key is in developing a consistent approach to eating that makes the food you eat work for you. I have learned how to combine my likes, dislikes, and common sense into a healthy weight-controlling food plan. It's an aware way of eating that I can enjoy and stick to for as long as I want. (Later in the book, I'll show how to make it work for you.)

So, quit casting yourself in the role of perennial loser. Get out of the self-defeating diet marathons. Prepare to set your own pace with an eating style that can make you look and feel like a winner every day.

4. Do you weigh in every morning, noon, and night?

Very often women hop on and off the scale regularly without realizing why. Most of the time it's a way to reinforce the no-win diet they're on or guilty about not being on. Don't kid yourself into thinking it's a progress check. Scale hoppers are more interested in measuring their failures than certifying their victories.

I used to keep a scale in almost every room of my apartment. There was even one in the corner of my living room. That scale allowed me to occasionally embarrass myself and entertain friends at the same time. I would get on the bathroom scale ten seconds after waking up in the morning. If the news was a bit better than I expected, I'd unconsciously eat more at breakfast and get back on the scale before I could squander an ounce. Now I had something tangible to worry about.

When you're worried about something you naturally pick at it. That means back again to the scales after lunch. One more time following coffee at three o'clock. Dinner called for a weigh-in before the melon and a weigh-out after the dietetic dessert. Come bedtime, I'd brush my teeth while stepping on the scale for a final blast. Try having sweet dreams with visions of extra pounds dancing in your head.

I told myself that the weigh-ins were for my own good. They would make me conscious of nibbling between meals or taking a portion larger than my diet allowed. The only thing the scale prevented was a self-assured ego. I needed a number check every few hours to decide how I felt about myself. I began to believe the numbers more than my own judgment. Ann Harper could deceive herself, but scales don't lie.

When the scale readings were up my mood was down. Sometimes the only way to cope with the scale was to get off the diet. Then I could console myself with a box of cookies and defy the scale to stop me. Of course, ending the diet only increased my use of the scale. How else could I compute the damage I was doing to myself?

A couple of years ago I threw away all my scales—except one. The lone surviving scale is buried deep in my hall closet. I dig it out once a month or so. But it's a big enough project to make me think about it at least twice. Usually I have to be in a pretty good mood to make that kind of effort. In essence, my scale has become a secondary success meter. It's a way of affirming the progress I already know I've made.

Scales were never meant to indicate how far from normal you are. That's a perversion we've added in the last twenty years. To hell with those weight charts stuck on pharmacy scales or tattooed to the cover of paperback diet books. How dare they give those chiseled-in-stone prescriptions for the perfect weight for a woman of such-and-such height. There is no single ideal weight for a 5-foot-6-inch woman. Even the charts that break things down into small, medium, and large frames fail to consider many essential factors.

A standard height-weight chart, plucked from a famous body-builders manual, mandates that 5-foot-6-inch women with large frames should be 146 pounds at most. They determine her frame by the size of her wrists. Heaven protect the broad-shouldered woman with slender wrists. She would be listed as a small-framed woman who had to weigh 123 pounds or less. My god, those shoulders would have to be resting on toothpick legs and no waist.

Your frame is more accurately determined by overall bone structure. Width of shoulders, pelvic bone, and chest cavity give a truer reading. Also, our all-knowing chart forgets to indicate how these pounds are distributed. If you're 146 pounds with a nonexistent bustline, you won't be nearly as attractive as a 180-pounder with a fully developed chest in proportion with broad hips and an ample derrière. Length of torso, waist, and legs should be considered, too. Basically, use your eyes, not their rigid gimmicks to categorize yourself.

By the way, none of these charts bothers to differentiate between a sixteen-year-old high school student and a mature woman of forty. Bodies do thicken with age, and the effect could be more sensual. The weight ranges also ignore how many children a woman has mothered. A thirty-year-old woman with three children deserves some leeway for what her body has been through.

Okay, let's throw away the charts and hide the scales. Instead of weighing in like clockwork, study the contour of your body. You should calculate any losses or gains by the way certain clothes fit. Find a dress that makes you look great. That's a goal that makes sense. When that size-18 dress hangs perfectly on you, real progress has been made. Until you reach that goal, keep an eye on how snug or loose your current size-20 outfits seem. That will cue you in to the daily ups and downs your weight is taking. Remember, people are watching you, not the numbers on your scale.

5. Do you act your age?

Relax, I'm not accusing you of acting like a child. Don't get offended—yet. Actually, I'm suggesting something a whole lot worse. Many large women unconsciously create the illusion of being older than they are. Your style of dress and carriage can appear to add as many as twenty years to your true age.

Do you confuse fuller-figure dimensions with having to be matronly? Maybe you do without fully realizing it. Evaluate your present image by stacking yourself up against skinnier, chic women of your own age bracket. When they wear designer jeans to a causal get-together, do you show up in a polyester pantsuit? At a disco-style party the crowd is decked out in sexy, high-slit skirts or clingy low-cut dresses. If you're the only one in a conservative A-line cover-all atrocity, then start looking for the fountain of youth.

The fashion industry was responsible for the fuller-figure granny complex in the past. Size 16s and over were expected to dress like they were seventy from the time they were teenagers. But you no longer can use that as your excuse. Smartly cut actionwear is now available for larger women of all ages. This allows you to pick and choose according to your years and the youthfulness of your spirit. Where there were only sixty manufacturers servicing large women's clothing needs five years ago, today we are catered to by over six hundred fashion-conscious firms.

Clothing is only part of the premature-aging dilemma. You can be dressed like a twelve-year-old gymnast, but let's see the way you move. Do you walk in short, mincing steps? Are you afraid to dance up a storm or trot after a bus or stride across a beach?

Only you really know how much you hold back. Be sensitive to your behavior in active situations. Your mind might be saying, "Heck, I'm too tired to do that now." But it may come out looking like you think you're too fat or maybe too *old*.

6. Do you limit yourself to spectator sports?

You're not exactly sure what I mean by "spectator sports." That's the name I give to games that you sit and watch, while others do the playing. It's another way of taking a matronly, self-defeating attitude toward your body. Oh, you might pretend to get involved in the contest. Your eyes follow the action and your voice cracks with enthusiasm. But the old body just hangs out in a blob.

Here's a description of the "interested spectator." If it sounds too familiar, then it's time to retrain your athletic ego. Our spectator is the large gal swiveling her head back and forth at a tennis match in the local park, cheering wildly for her office mates at the co-ed softball game, and pressing her nose to the chalet window as girl friends ski briskly down the slope. She is the sideline heroine who gets to hold everybody's jewelry, keeps an eye on the coats, and never misses a turn as scorekeeper. She's also the official soda lady, cocoa getter, sandwich maker. When the game is over, she seems to feel all the agony of defeat without ever experiencing the exhilaration of competing.

That's you? Too bad. I'm afraid you tend to see yourself as the stereotypical "fat nonathlete." It's a complex stemming from the vicious myth about fuller-figure women being less graceful, alert, coordinated, and competitive than skinnier women of the same age. Honestly, it's not true! Unfortunately, you'll continue to accept this distortion until you put on your sneakers and prove to yourself how wrong it is.

As a young teenager, I was hesitant to do anything that would draw attention to my body. I alternated between being a Sideline Sadie and a reluctant participant. There were times when my ego took a battering. I botched an easy grounder in softball, couldn't reach drop volleys in tennis, and felt like a snowbound walrus after losing a ski in a snowdrift. However, once I got over my own disasters I noticed how everybody else managed to trip up in their own special way. The laugh wasn't always on me.

By my mid-twenties, I was fairly good at the sports I cared about. More importantly I had been enjoying them for years. Practice was the key to both. Trying over and over makes the big difference for a size-28 novice, just like it does for a size-6 beginner. The shame is that the size-28 woman was always afraid of abuse and failure. Meanwhile, Spunky Ms. Size 6 was guaranteed encouragement and a shot at success. Luckily, it's never too late to get into the game.

Make sure you start your sporting days with the right attitude. Big women can be graceful and effective athletes. Top tennis star Betty Stover is six feet tall and quite husky, yet she moves and volleys with the absolute best women professionals in the world. Several fuller-figure women won gold medals at the Olympics, and the girth of world-class women athletes in general is growing bigger every year.

Anyhow, you're not taking up a sport to win world championships or cop coveted medals. Don't worry about how well you play at first. The idea is to enjoy yourself, meet people, and shape up the body. Take some group lessons in the individual sports, like tennis, golf, skiing, and squash. The instructor will give you the proper basics to guarantee that you'll look and play as competently as possible. The group will start you off in the company of other newcomers. They'll be glad to give you the kind of support they themselves are looking for.

Team sports shouldn't be ignored either.

Really, what could be more fantastic than joining a mixed softball, bowling or volleyball team? You have games and available men all together in a foam of beer parties (light beer of course), team spirit, and good-natured fun. Also, you don't have to be the Atomic Flash in these games. In softball and volleyball you are assigned a position to cover, and that's it. Stick to your sort and try hard. The rest is fate, fun, and learning the ropes.

I know there are some sports you just can't bring yourself to try. That's perfectly normal. Nobody even claims to have attempted them all. I swim, bicycle, play tennis, and ski cross-country and downhill. In addition, I take dance classes in tap and jazz whenever I can. But to this day I don't dare to put on water skis. I probably never will.

So, when all my friends water ski, I'm the interested—from a distance—spectator. I comfortably curl up under a beach umbrella and soak in their falls rather than the sun. That's okay, since I know that I don't *limit* myself to purely spectator sports.

7. Are you talking the wrong body language?

Saying that you feel confident, graceful, and at ease with yourself is not enough. At times your body communicates a different message. It takes a trained eye to hear what your anatomy is saying about itself. You have to learn the language of your body before you can be sure it's speaking about you in positive terms.

When you meet a group of people for the first time, does your body speak up proudly? Think about it! Too many large women act as if they're ashamed of their bulk. They believe that a hunched-over, quiet, low profile will keep strangers from clearly noticing just how big they are. These women psychologically shrink themselves by acting demure. Yet, as their own self-esteem dwindles, their physique looms larger and more evident.

What's worse, many fuller-figure ladies greet new aquaintances with their eyes cast downward. Do you suddenly get too facinated with your shoes at a party? That's almost like whispering, "I'm not good enough for you." The least it tells the other person is that you're too self-conscious about something to make eye contact. Meeting another stare openly is a way of touching somebody casually as an equal. It shows a willingness to make a friendly, honest exchange.

I suggest you enter a room slowly with your chin up. Keep your manner strong with an air of confidence. That doesn't mean stiff as a board! Walk around with a preset course in mind. False starts will only make your weight seem awkward. It's necessary for your body to state plainly, "I don't have to make excuses for being a big gal."

On the other hand, don't confuse being secure about your body with the overly aggressive stance some big women activists have been recommending lately. Big doesn't have to come across as awesome. There's no need to barge into a room breathing fire. You only hurt yourself by cowing people with your presence. Any figure that totally dominates a scene tends to invite more negative than positive comments.

Your personality shouldn't be altered too drastically by your size. The language your body speaks must consistently seem natural and appropriate for the woman you are. Subtlely let yourself find the tone of your surroundings. You do fit in!

8. Is it better to give and never receive?

Your common sense may be arguing, "No, only a fair give-and-take is tolerable." But check to see if your actions back up that opinion. Large women are notorious for compulsively giving more to others than they ever hope to get in return. Some of us develop this doormat approach to relationships as a way of assuring acceptance from groups or individuals we're fond of. We almost beg these people to take advantage of us.

How many times have you faithfully watered this neighbor's plants when she was away? Or spent two weeks caring for that neighbor's sick cat while he went off to play in the Caribbean? But during your vacation the greenery in your living room turned to brown. Your prized ferns withered from total neglect. And your omnipresent pussycat yowled for five hundred miles in the back seat of the car.

Or perhaps you're the dependable mother forever posted outside the schoolyard gate at three o'clock. Every Monday through Friday you're waiting to pick up your daughter and seven other people's kids. Then Jenny's mother isn't home and Eric's mom just has an errand or two to do. Well, the children are at your house already! After all you're such an angel.

Hang your halo up for a rest. You're a person with feelings just like anybody else. Don't continue to make two dishes for the weekly

card game, especially if you end up alone in a friend's kitchen cleaning up. Practice saying no to demeaning requests. I know it's not so easy. But the few favors you do will mean more when people know they have to be earned with mutual concern.

I learned that lesson the hard way when I first got into modeling. Back in the early seventies, I was the only fuller-figure woman working the major ads. It made me think of myself as the Jolly Green Giant in the Valley of the Dolls. Somehow, I decided that the other models would accept my size easier if I bent over backward to be accomodating.

The extremes I went to for their approval! Frequently, I'd come early for a booking to put in extra time on my makeup. When the skinnies arrived I'd retreat to a corner of the dressing room to allow them to spread out their belongings. See how little space I take up? Next, I'd volunteer to get lunch for the photographer, models, and crew. Why, I'd even make it a habit to drop a couple of the models off after the shooting in a taxi I paid for. They never reciprocated.

Why should they? I held my kindness so cheaply. It wasn't until my second year in the business that I felt secure enough to treat the other models as equals. It worked beautifully! When I did a favor for one of the girls, it was out of affection or appreciation. Top fashion stars like Vibeke and Franziska sensed my self-esteem and became more complimentary and giving. I never again felt forced into being nice.

The one-sided relationships you're in are probably with people who really want to show concern for you. Most likely they're waiting for a sign. We all respond to somebody who openly commands our respect. So stop trying to compensate for your big body by treating yourself as less of a person. Set an example for friends to follow. Be positively big and proud and love the one you're always with—YOU!

Did you pass the quiz? Don't bother counting how many yeses or nos you put down. It's not a matter of browbeating yourself either. The only criterion for a high score is how you *now* think of yourself. Do you want to make the most of your *real* size, age, grace, and other assets? A yes here makes you a fuller-figure genius.

Once you have a Big Beauty self-image you are ready to go to work on your body. Begin by focusing your eyes, adjusting your glasses, or cleaning those contact lenses. You're about to get an overview of yourself from top to toe that will pop your pupils. Each part of your body will be identified as a viable type with a presence all its own.

CHAPTER THREE

BALANCING YOUR BODY

A while ago I was booked to do a lingerie ad for a silky, rather sheer undergarment called a teddy. The one-piece teddy was always considered too sexy or playful for us fuller-figure women. But I knew after one hard glance that I looked great in it. All the negative and positive aspects of my body seemed to be balanced out by the way the teddy was cut.

In the full-length mirror I could see that my large head appeared smaller when more of my figure was revealed. Left bare, my broad shoulders came across as a lot less over-powering, yet they were still wide enough to offset the fullness of my hips and thighs. The V-shaped lacework in the midsection of the teddy created an illusion of a smaller waistline,

which made me look even more like a figure 8 than usual. And uncovering my whole leg elongated my meaty thighs, emphasized my shapely calves, even drew attention to my proverbial "well-turned" ankles.

Knowing how to evaluate your body is a must for every professional model. It enables us to always give a well-proportioned, confident appearance. You don't have to be a model, however, to get in touch with the curves and angles that form your figure. I can show you an easy-to-understand method for categorizing each part of your body. Ultimately, you will use this information to select the styles best suited to your dimensions.

Please don't expect to make an on-the-spot

appraisal of your pluses and minuses by merely gazing into a mirror. This isn't a bit of the queen's magic taken from the pages of Snow White. The quick study I did of myself was the product of years of preparation. I talked with many beauty experts, pored over thousands of pictures, got feedback from other models, *and* stood in front of mirrors for hours.

Your insights will come from dissecting some carefully posed photographs of yourself. But first you'll have to do a few simple things. Get the help of a cooperative friend. Make sure you have a trustworthy camera. Keep a log or notebook handy to jot down what you've learned. Follow my directions to the letter for taking yourself apart. And smile— it's completely painless!

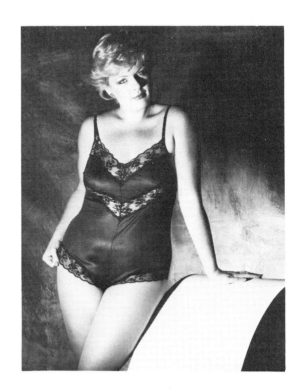

GETTING THE PICTURE

You can begin by making a list of the shots you will need for your head-to-toe analysis. There must be two frontal full-body photos. One will be in a leotard and the other in street clothes. Next, you should get a total profile shot also taken in a leotard. Finally, zero in for a pair of shoulders-up head shots that capture the features of your face. I strongly suggest that you take several shots of each pose or perhaps get hold of an instant-developing camera.

Try to wear the same color tights and leotard for the first full-length shot. When your body is a monotone, those hard-to-gauge trouble spots, such as the thighs, won't appear heavier just because your tights are a lighter shade. However, you do want the leotards and tights to contrast sharply with the backdrop. An all-white or pale wall allows you to clearly see where and how much work is required.

You should stand up straight with your back to the wall. That doesn't mean up against the wall! We want to avoid any leaning, which tends to throw the picture off. Distribute your weight evenly on feet spread about ten to twelve inches apart. Let your arms dangle loosely at your sides. Relax. Then make sure your friend is shooting from far enough away to get every lovely inch of you into the eye of the camera.

In the second shot wear the clothes you had on to go shopping the other day. Don't whip up something special for the occasion. Again stand in front of the wall facing the camera. By closely examining this snapshot later, we'll be able to see how many of your figure problems are corrected by the way you now dress. It will also point out which flaws your present wardrobe only makes worse.

For the profile photo stand sideways with your shoulder a few inches away from the pale wall. Keep your feet together this time. Hold your back and shoulders upright, but in a manner that goes along with your normal posture. Once more, place your hands at your sides. The purpose of the profile is to highlight the contour of your body. Here we see exactly where you're ripely round or firmly flat. A word of caution: Asking your friend to gently shake the camera while shooting won't solve anything.

Both head shots should be done identically. Start by pulling your curls or bangs back in the front to expose the hairline. Use a tight headband to hold your hair securely. Then have your photographer take full-face shots. Aim to fill up as much of the picture as possible without losing the complete outline of the head. Your neck and shoulder tops are slightly less important to us in this situation. The head shots will be used later to determine, among other things, the shape of your face and the size of your forehead.

That's the end of your shooting session. The photographs you've taken freeze for inspection all the physical sides of you the rest of the world sees every day. Not totally thrilled with the results? Don't worry! You are about to cut them up into tidy pieces with your trusty ballpoint pen.

TAKING YOURSELF APART

One of your prime concerns is to measure how well the various parts of your body relate to each other. What areas of your physique dominate a passerby's attention? Which features wind up being overwhelmed? We can begin to find the answers by dividing you into four visual sections.

Front View

Take out the frontal photograph of you in the leotard and tights. Okay, let's do a little pen-and-ink cosmetic surgery. Draw a scalpel-fine line across the base of the neck. Put another line through your natural waistline—that refers to the contour of your midsection, not where you might buckle a low-slung belt. Finish off with a third slash over the top of the legs.

The picture now defines your standard beauty zones. Head: top of scalp to bottom

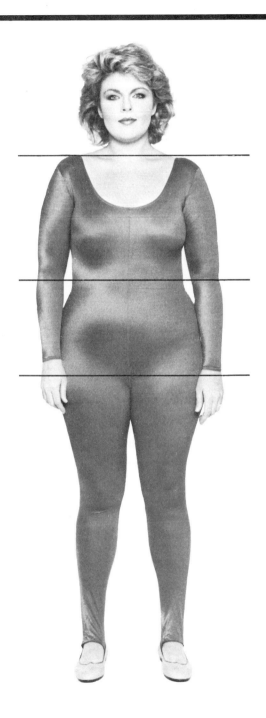

of the neck. Upper torso: shoulders to waistline. Lower torso: waistline down to where the thighs begin. Legs: thighs all the way to tips of toes. Each zone represents approximately a quarter of your total look. On a perfectly proportioned woman each zone catches the eye equally.

The easiest and most direct way to categorize your body is to start from the top. How large is your head? Look at the whole photo first. Decide if the head appears to fit your body well. If it *seems* insignificant in comparison to your upper torso, then write down that your head is *small for body*. If your head tends to dwarf your upper torso, then mark it *large for body*. When your head comfortably shares attention with your upper torso, it should be termed *average for body*. Later on, I'll provide tips for making your head appear either larger or more delicate.

Now, on the same frontal photo, pen in vertical lines running from each shoulder down to either side of your waistline. Then, continue the vertical lines on down until they meet the horizontal line at the top of your legs. You have enclosed your upper and lower torso in two distinct boxes. These boxes make it simpler to visually analyze your figure.

Ideally, the upper torso and lower torso should be equal. However, if the upper-torso box is shorter than the lower torso box, you are obviously *short-waisted*. When the upper box is longer it indicates that you're *long-waisted*. Don't forget to note your findings in the log. In the chapter entitled "Fuller-Figure Fashion: A Brave New World," I'll show you how to alter your waistline so that it falls in just the right spot.

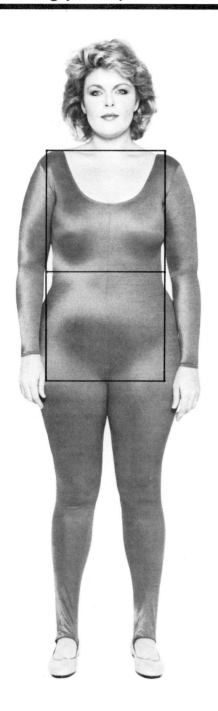

Grab your pen again. Go over the outer borders of both the upper- and lower-torso boxes. This should give you a darkened rectangle that includes the whole torso region. Then, form a second rectangle by sketching lines down from the hip joints (at top of the legs) to a horizontal line at your toes. You can now readily compare your leg zone to your torso.

Do the two rectangles seem to be of equal length? A yes means you can say you're in *perfect overall proportion lengthwise*. If the torso rectangle is shorter, then you can call yourself *leggy*. A longer upper rectangle informs you that you're *short-legged*. Fashion pointers will also cover ways of coping with different leg lengths.

Side View

The profile photograph will give us a chance to see how robust your curves are—front and back. Take pen in hand and draw a vertical line from the corner of your shoulder (middle of arm-shoulder joint) straight down the center of your side to the floor. This will divide your profile into a front half and back half. Follow up by dissecting it with a horizontal line at the waist. Your figure and the picture are now broken down into quadrants.

Number the upper left-hand corner of the photo *1*. Put a *2* in the upper-right corner, a *3* in the bottom left and a *4* in the bottom-right corner. We'll use these numbers as a convenient method of identifying the quadrants. You might want to diagram the photo and corresponding numbers into your notebook as an added reference.

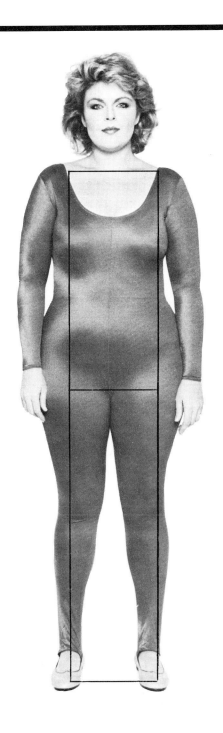
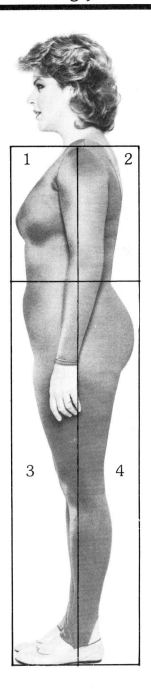

Study the photograph closely. Do you think your chest fills about as much of quadrant 1 as your derriere does of quadrant 4? A yes answer suggests you're *balanced*. If the chest takes up decisively more of its quadrant, then label yourself *top heavy*. But if your rear blocks out more of quadrant 3, then you must consider yourself *bottom heavy*. Easy, it's not the end of the world! Just calmly record the findings under the diagram in your log. I have some great equalizers for you in the chapter on clothing.

All right, let's pull a couple of additional views from the profile photo. Carefully estimate if your tummy bulges into quadrant 3 as far as your chest protrudes into quadrant 1. Getting a fix on your stomach will help you to eventually select the right style of skirt. Then see if your backside takes up as much of quadrant 4 as your belly does of its quadrant. I'll be using this information to put you into the right kind of pants or jeans for your torso. Remember, an overbearing posterior is seen as *full*, a moderate fanny is called *round*, and a nonexistent one is universally known as *flat-ended*.

WHOLE-BODY TYPES

Clinically picking yourself apart made it easier to identify specific body facts and failings. Now, by utilizing some of what you've learned, I'll show you how to get yourself back together again. Actually, I'll be helping you to classify yourself as a whole-body type. Each type suggests an overall contour for your physique. It gives an overview of how you're proportioned.

Each whole-body type calls for a different general fashion philosophy.

Spread out your marked-up frontal and profile shots on the table. We'll be using them as a visual aid. Also, keep the log handy for notes on what kind of fuller figure you have. Here are the four major whole body types: Figure 8, pear shape, barrel shape, and box shape. Which one fits you best?

Figure 8

This is the shape of the famous femme fatales. Mae West vamped her way through decades by throwing around her so-called hourglass figure. Marilyn Monroe made calendars into popular art by undressing her figure 8 over the dates. Beverly Sills visually earned her nickname "Bubbles" by cutting a classic form on the opera stage. Even Yours Truly managed to create some sexy pictures thanks to my full figure 8.

The figure-8 design is considered to be the most evenly proportioned of the large-woman body types. On the frontal photograph the upper-torso box is a perfect match for the lower-torso box. There is also a visible indentation at your waistline. A red pen should be able to start at your broad shoulders, swing around an ample chest, across a slightly pinched waist, and over a wide hip, before doing an inverted S back to the shoulders. In most cases, the legs are equal in length to the torso.

Women who are lucky enough to have this shape will find future shopping a pleasure. Almost anything can fit into your wardrobe. Very few figure corrections are required. But

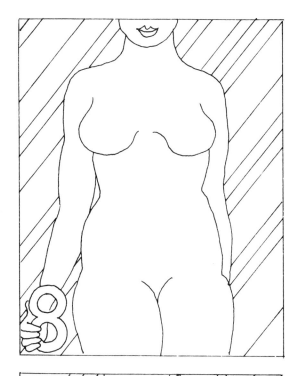

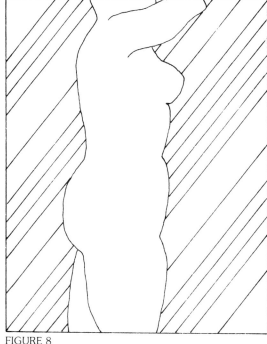

FIGURE 8

I'll show you ways of turning every figure 8 into a peerless "10."

Pear Shape

The pear shape is great for diamonds and fruit lovers. Unfortunately, it can cause chronic fashion headaches for many large women. Those of you who fall into this category pretty much know who you are. You're the ones walking around with perhaps a size-14 upper torso centered over maybe a size-20 lower torso.

Examine the frontal photo one more time. The lower box is noticeably wider than the upper torso box. Generally, the lower torso bells out into the thigh section. On the profile shots you saw that you were obviously bottom-heavy. Yet, your rather wide hips do give you the illusion of a fine waistline. A red pencil could vividly outline the pear shape if you traced around your torso from knees to neck and back again.

I know it appears to be a bleak glamour situation. What can you possibly wear? Well, there is a whole variety of styles that can cure your fashion woes. Mixing and matching lives!

Barrel Shape

Sound like more trouble than a keg of dynamite? Please don't start imagining people rolling you over and over down an endless hill. Women with a barrel shape tend to have quite a few physical blessings and only a minor curse or two. However, very few women know how to recognize a barrel figure.

According to the frontal photograph, your

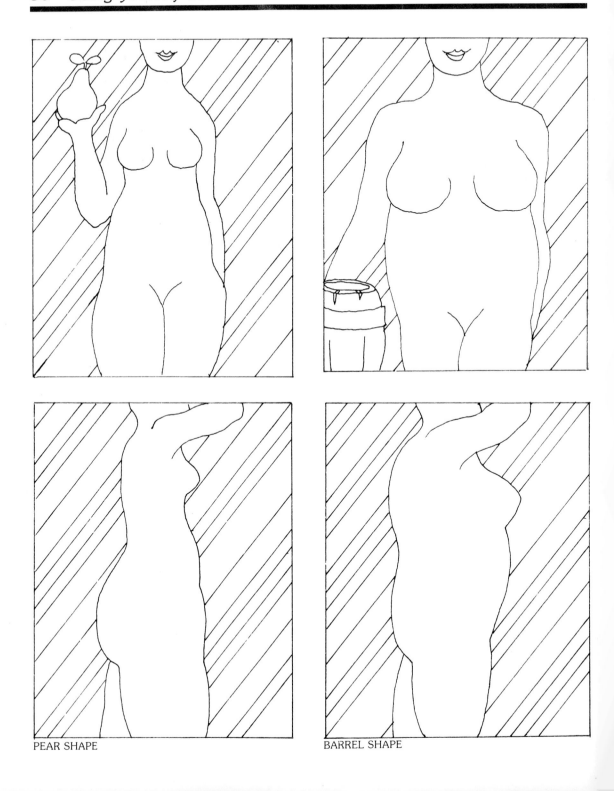

PEAR SHAPE

BARREL SHAPE

upper torso seems to be short, but broader than the lower torso. This translates into being short-waisted and wide-shouldered. In the profile you're profoundly top-heavy, which explains the term *barrel-chested*. However, you surprisingly come up light in the caboose. Yes, you're absolutely flat-ended.

A big problem for the barrel-shape woman is her waist. You're probably thicker in the middle than you are at the hips. Barrels do bulge, you know! But don't pout about it too long. Most of you also have fantastically slender thighs and a great pair of gams.

Box Shape

This is another way of saying fully firm and evenly packed. Women with a box shape are broad all around, straight up and down. They're enclosed by wide lines or right angles. Curves just never seem to come into the picture.

A peek at the frontal shot gives you the facts squarely in the eye. The upper torso and lower torso are equal in *every* direction. Yet, unlike the figure 8, there is no visible waistline. You are simply one unbroken box from shoulders to hips. Fortunately, most of your figure flaws can be solved by artificially manufacturing an indented waistline for you. I'll be throwing some curves your way in the fashion chapter.

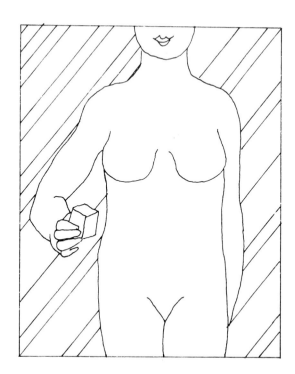

Face shapes

The first and last word in any beauty analysis has to be about your face. This is where your personality, emotions, and intellect combine with your physical features. Eyes always focus

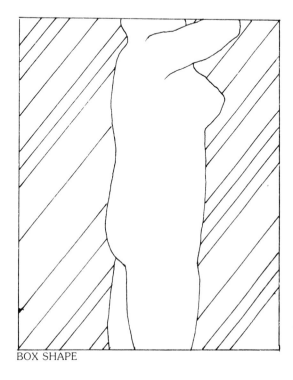

BOX SHAPE

on your face before scanning the rest of your body. It's an expected reflex action.

Regrettably, many women work at putting together a gorgeous face without really seeing themselves clearly. Sure, you're aware of things like the color of your eyes or the size of your nose. Yet, you can't accurately describe the overall shape of your face. What is the geometric appearance created by tracing the cut of your jawline, the cheekbone angles, the expanse of your forehead? Don't just avoid the question! The answer is essential for choosing truly flattering makeup techniques, hairstyles, or facial accessories.

Using one of the head shots you took earlier as a worksheet, darken the borders of your face by running a pen from the middle of your hairline all the way around the jawline —excluding the ears—and back up again. Now, match this outline of your face to one of the following descriptions. There are six basic face shapes: oval, round, square, diamond, triangle, and heart. Some of you might see yourself as a combination of two different shapes. Don't panic! I'm half heart and half square, myself.

Oval

The "ultimate oval" is the model's, artist's, or photographer's dream. Every aspect of the oval face is in perfect proportion. The forehead, cheeks, and chin are all in balance. There are no sharp angles, just delicately curving lines forming a slender oval shape.

Round

The round face has a much broader total look than the oval. But, like the oval shape, there are no hard angles in the cheeks or jawline. The cheeks are simply quite wide. In fact, if you subdivided the round face into quadrants, all parts would be equal. People with round faces also tend to have wide, short foreheads.

Square

These faces are highlighted by their prominent, angular jaws—you know, the kind of jaws that are supposed to promise strong convictions. The width of the jaw seems to be about the same as the forehead. Meanwhile, the cheekbones are wide-set and sharp enough to give a high, classy impression.

Diamond

Diamond-shaped faces are all pointy in the key areas. They are reminiscent of the baseball diamond, not the little gems lodged in your jewelry. Draw a straight line from the middle of the hairline to each cheek, then from the cheeks to the center of the chin. With your chin as home plate, take a dash around the bases to see if the diamond fits the face. You take off from a chin that narrows to almost a point. The face gradually angles out to a wide left cheek (first base), before starting to edge inward again to a narrow forehead (second). Once more the path darts wide to the right cheek (third base) prior to closing in on the chin. Some women like to think of it as a sharper version of the oval.

Triangle

These faces start off on top like the diamond shape, except in this instance everything just keeps angling outward. The forehead here is as narrow as it was in the diamond face. Then

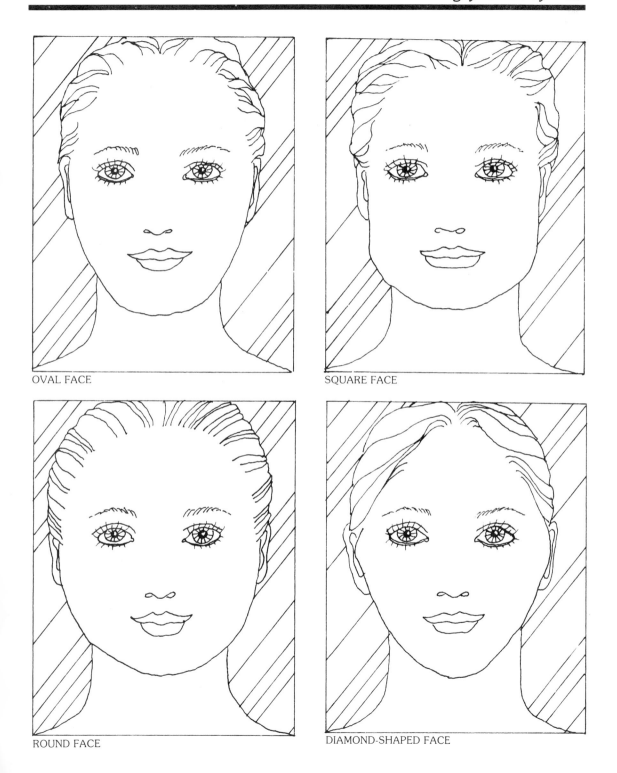

OVAL FACE

SQUARE FACE

ROUND FACE

DIAMOND-SHAPED FACE

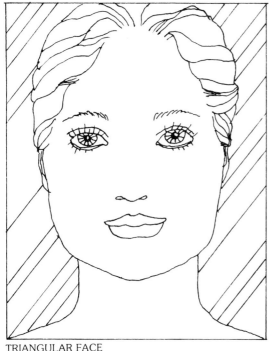

TRIANGULAR FACE

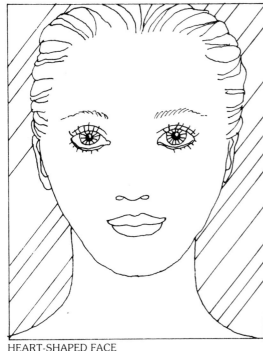

HEART-SHAPED FACE

the cheekbones jut out a bit wider than the forehead. Next, the jawline expands out past the edge of the cheeks. Finally, a broad chin combines with the jawline to create a solid, quite horizontal-looking foundation. You could say it has a certain amount of pyramid power.

Heart

When you read the description, heart-shaped faces sound like upside-down triangles. However, the line you drew around the perimeter on your photograph definitely forms a heart. The forehead is fairly wide and rounds into a slightly narrower cheek area on each side. These cheekbones slope down to a jawline that converges into a relatively pointed chin. The only thing that's missing is Cupid's arrow.

Your face shape should be recorded in the ongoing log. I think it would be wise to list all the features of your face's outline on the same page. Remember to emphasize where your characteristics deviate from a basic face shape.

By the way, there is one more observation that could be added at this time. Your forehead's length is as much of a factor in glamorizing the face as is the width. It figures in both the shape and proportions of your face.

To see what kind of forehead you're working with, turn to the second head shot. Divide your face into thirds by drawing horizontal lines across the arch of the eyebrows and under the tip of the nose. If the top third is longer than the bottom two areas, you boast a *high forehead*. Conversely, you have a *low forehead*, if the upper facial section is the

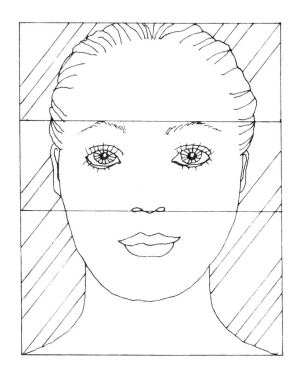

shortest. When all three portions are exactly even, you are considered to have an *average-length forehead*.

Okay, soul mates, the introductions are over! We've shared some common experiences, pondered our self-images, and become better acquainted with our bodies. What you need is some rapid-fire glamour tips. The next part of the book gives you dozens of dramatic make-overs that will make you visibly prettier right away. Get ready to put all the notes you've scribbled down to practical use.

PART TWO

INSTANT GLAMOUR:

HEAD-TO-TOE

BEAUTY QUICKIES

CHAPTER FOUR

MAKEUP:

FACIAL ILLUSIONS

When was the last time you worked make-up magic on your face? Think it over. I don't see anything magical about caking on a heavy foundation that's topped off with random colors. Adding false eyelashes or pale lipstick won't turn the beauty trick, either. Too many large women just hide behind a cosmetic veil.

Making up is a lot more than merely covering up. A really good makeup job creates several attractive and slenderizing illusions. Other people see your face as glamourously improved. They're busy marveling at your beautiful features rather than commenting on your cosmetic skills. The makeup becomes part of your natural look.

Actually, it's amazing how many facial problems you can zap away with a little makeup know-how. For instance, your close-set eyes can suddenly appear to be wider apart. A slightly crooked nose can be viewed as perfectly centered. Those embarrassing double chins may seem to vanish. Even your short, thick neck could now give a deceivingly slimmer impression.

I know, you're wondering about how hard it must be to apply makeup this effectively. Well, it's similar to learning any other kind of magic. Making up only looks difficult to the outsider. Once you're shown how to do the tricks, it becomes very easy. Then you just pick the right illusions for your face and begin to use them.

Trust me! Give up the old makeup routines

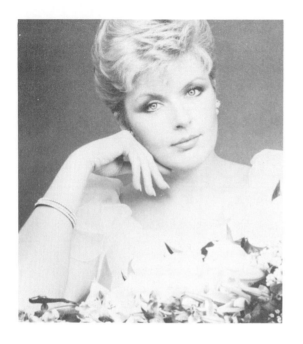

you got too comfortable with as a kid. Bring your face into the present. You don't have to keep the same face for your whole adult life. Facial images should change almost as often as hairstyles or the latest Paris fashions—well, maybe not quite that quickly. But what have you got to lose? If the face you try doesn't wow you, simply wash it down the drain.

As a model I'm always searching for a new look. In fact, I periodically spend whole days doing nothing but *testing*. At a test session I'll team up with a makeup artist and beauty photographer to experiment with different faces. The artist uses my face as an erasable canvas for his ideas and, from selecting the appropriate cosmetics through the finished picture, it's always a complete learning situation for me.

I watch to see what tools, brushes, and pencils the various makeup experts prefer. After a while, the colors and techniques for application become familiar, and I find myself anticipating the artist's next move, even their use of lighting. Later, I can check to see how the whole thing stands up to the photographer's harsher lights. Here's where superior highlighting and contouring methods really show.

In my decade of modeling I've done hundreds of exciting test sessions and seen top artists do just about every beauty trick that can benefit the face of a fuller-figure woman. Now, I'm ready to pass along the best of these trade secrets to you. For your own test session I'll give you everything you need to conjure up a new, beautifully balanced, thinner-looking face. Then, a highly respected makeup magician will help guide you through

Makeup: facial illusions **41**

three fantastic make-overs: a basic daytime look, a five-minute emergency face, and the ultraglamorous evening face.

Ready? Let's start from scratch. Open your notebooks to a clean page and write down the information that specifically applies to you. Believe me, you'll have plenty of valuable tips to remember.

TOOLS OF THE MAKEUP TRADE

Even Houdini needed the correct props to make his illusions convincing. Your makeup magic requires a modest collection of simple gadgets, brushes, and soft goods. However, don't buy everything a professional makeup artist uses. Cut some financial corners. For example, a costly set of brushes is an unnecessary expense. Pick and choose the brushes you'll really need. Then buy them individually.

Before doing any shopping take inventory of the makeup equipment you already own. On a sheet of paper headed "What I Have," list the usable items. Later, in a column on the same page entitled "What I Need," write down the tools I recommend. This will prevent the extra outlay for doubles of a certain thing.

By the way, most of the brushes and devices mentioned in this section can be found in one of the following places:

☐ A beauty supply house carrying a large cosmetic stock.

☐ Makeup specialty stores—check local Yellow Pages.

☐ An art-supply store.

Beware! Clerks sometimes get too zealous in their sales pitch. Go in there with a shopping list; come out with only the essentials.

The tool box

GADGETS

tweezers (get slant-edged or pointed; avoid flat-edged type because you could easily tweeze out too many hairs)

eyelash curlers

two pencil sharpeners (one large enough for fat shadow pencils and a small one for lip pencils)

BRUSHES

1/8-inch flat artist's brush (measured by width; for blending)

two 1/4-inch flat artist's brushes (for blending around eyes)

four dry-powder-shadow brushes (a narrow one for each color you might use)

small rounded paintbrush (very soft sable bristles for powdering eyelids)

large powder brush (also soft; for powdering whole face)

three soft cosmetic blush brushes (a small tapered contour brush for specific spots and two regular-sized brushes)

slant-edged lip brushes (two with stiff bristles)

SOFT GOODS

A hand towel (place on cosmetic table beneath tools; also to wipe excess color from brushes—paper tears too easily)

bottle of sterile alcohol (for cleaning tools at least once a week; always when sharing tools with a friend)

tissues

Q-tips (buy a large box)

makeup sponges (packages of three; cut into quarters for convenience; to wipe away excess foundation or color washes)

sponge-tipped shadow applicators (for putting on and blending certain eyeshadows; put into alcohol and use over and over)

CHOOSING YOUR COSMETICS

Your beautiful new face will be a subtle mixture of colors, textures, and highlights. Each person's face requires a slightly different combination of makeups to achieve the best possible results. You must take into consideration your skin tone, how dry or oily your skin happens to be, and even the color of your eyes. Yet, with a little thought and my advice, you'll have no trouble compiling a personal makeup kit.

First of all, get out of the neighborhood drugstore and go to the vast department stores, which very often have a much better choice of cosmetics. Also, the people working the various areas tend to know more about skin types and makeup in general. Don't hesitate to try on makeups or pump the employees for information.

Watch out for extremely high-priced brands pushed by chic specialty stores. Most of them are just not worth it. There are only a few large "powder houses" in this country. They make all the powder items (transluscent powder, blushes, sparkle dust, *et cetera*) for the cosmetic houses. It's most often the packaging and advertising that separates the cheaper brands from the more expensive ones. The quality is universally pretty much the same.

All right, now let's put together your cosmetic shopping list. I'll be telling you what to get in the order of application. Where it's appropriate, make sure you consult the color charts before making a purchase. Only buy the colors that compliment your particular face. Later, you can add seasonal colors as they become available. These embellish existing colors; they don't replace them.

The makeup kit

YOUR EYES

Eyeshadow base comes in a tube. Makes it easier to spread the various colors on your eyes.

EYESHADOW-POWDER COLORS

eye color	main shadow	highlighter
brown	rust, plum, gray, taupe (stay away from pastels)	pink, beige, peach
blue	gray, plum, lavender, rust	peach, pink
green/hazel	brown, plum, tawny, rust, taupe	peach, beige
gray/black	pink, lavender, plum	pink, peach

(Don't get all colors in your category. Select your favorites!)

Fat black pencil is an important part of eye makeup. Defines lids, helps shape eyes, and creates shadows.

Eyeshadow powders are much better than creams for large women. Creams melt off and get stuck in the creases of our eyes when we perspire. Buy a main eyeshadow powder and a paler one that acts as a highlighter. See chart for eyeshadow hues best for you.

Mascara is sold plain or with tiny particles. Particles give a lash-lengthening illusion and are fine for women with short lashes

Eyebrow pencil should be a shade lighter than your hair.

PREFOUNDATION LIQUIDS

Glycerine is used as a moisturizer before contouring.

Color correctors are liquids you apply to your skin prior to the foundation. Color correctors even out skin tone and get rid of color flaws. Examine chart to see which color corrector remedies a discoloration you may have.

color correctors	skin problem solved
yellow	corrects ruddy or very red skin (most common among large ladies)
violet	neutralizes blotches on pale and mildly sallow skin
peach	enlivens very sallow skin
red	evens out ashy blotches on black skin

THE FOUNDATION

Basic or overall foundation comes in either a moisturizing variety for dry skin or a water-base type for oily and combination skin. (See Chapter 5 for how to determine your skin type.) The water base foundation won't perspire during a pressure-packed situation or tense moment. Check the foundation color chart to find the best shade for your skin.

Contour is a darker layer of foundation than your skin tone. Consult foundation color chart.

Opaque concealer creme is easier to apply than concealers sold in a tube, should be lighter than your skin shade, and can be used as a highlighter. See foundation color chart.

Yellow concealer is sometimes referred to as Mellow Yellow. It is used to cover red blemishes or enlarged capillaries. These skin spots are common problems for large women. Dab on the yellow concealer before applying the basic foundation and you'll never see red again.

POWDERS

Baby powder absorbs liquids and "sets" makeup.

Translucent powder is manufactured by cosmetic companies and sold loose or compressed in compacts. The loose variety gives more setting power when used on a foundation and also comes with sparkles; save this for evening makeup.

BLUSHERS

Color washes are relatively new to the beauty industry. Great for times when you don't want to use a foundation. Color washes work like a diluted rouge and can look very natural.

Blush powders perk up your complexion and make you look a little healthier. There are

FOUNDATION COLORS*

skin tone	basic/overall	contour	opaque concealer
light	light	medium	light
medium	medium	dark	light
dark	medium	dark	medium
red	yellow beige	dark	medium
yellow	rose beige	warm medium	light
bronze	bronze	dark	bronze
ash black	warm dark	none	warm dark
true black	warm dark	none	warm medium

*If you have difficulty determining your skin tone, consult a cosmetician. When choosing a foundation color, hair color should also be taken into consideration. A woman with darker hair can get away with stronger colors for her face.

BLUSH COLORS

skin tone	main	accent	blending
light	mauve	pink	pink
medium	rust	coral	pink
dark	wine	plum	pink
red	bronze	rust	coral
yellow	mauve	pink	lavender
bronze	coral	rose	pink
ash black	plum	wine	none
true black	red	purple	coral

LIP COLORS

skin tone	lip colors
light	pink, plum, or clear red
medium	rust, coral, or clear red
dark	wine, plum, or red
red	rust or coral
yellow	red or plum
bronze	coral, rose, or bronze
ash black	plum or wine
true black	red, plum, wine, or pink

three kinds of blushers that you'll need. First, a slightly darker *main blusher*. Next, a brightly colored *accent*. And finally, a paler blusher for *blending*. These powders are usually pressed into compacts, and the colors should once again be matched to your skin tone.

LIPSMACKERS

Flesh-colored lip pencil defines the shape of your lips.

Lipsticks are preferable to other forms of lip colors. Get two or three lipsticks for variety.
Lip gloss comes in tubes, pots, and sticks. Goes over lipstick to create shiny, fuller lips.

IN THE RIGHT LIGHT

What you see in the mirror isn't always what you get! Many women are gorgeous in the bathroom mirror and turn surprisingly discolored by the time they reach the street. Don't threaten to sue the cosmetics companies. You just put your makeup on in the wrong light. The ideal situation is to sit facing the clear light of day. This way you get an absolutely trustworthy reflection. Most other kinds of lighting distort the true colors of your makeup. Even the amount of makeup you're wearing gets hard to determine. For example, flourescent lights drown out red and warm tones, while throwing off a green or bluish tint. You might as well be making up under water.

I know you can't always set things up so that you're facing daylight. Makeup goes on at all hours, and windows aren't necessarily right in front of you. However, I can show you how to devise some permanent and dependable alternatives that are simple to work out. And soon your indoor makeup nook will be bright as day at the snap of a switch.

LIGHTING ALTERNATIVES FOR MAKEUP

Set up a table on the wall *opposite a window*. You'll be sitting with your back to the window, but a mirror on the table will reflect the natural daylight on to your face. This won't 'be enough light, because your body will be partially in the way, so add two lamps that stand at the level of your face. Make sure they have plain shades. An unshaded bulb permits a harsh glare to bounce off the mirror.

Don't despair if you're stuck at a table *without any available daylight*. Simply attach makeup lights around the top and sides of your mirror. *Never* have lights beaming up from beneath your face. This will cause some

of the ugliest shadows you've ever seen. Furthermore, I don't endorse those makeup mirrors that claim to reflect every different kind of lighting. They're just not very effective.

Some of you must make up *in the bathroom*. Well, here it helps to be handy or have a handyman around the house. Install one incandescent fixture on either side of the medicine-cabinet mirror. Make sure they're at the height of your face while peering into the mirror. You can use two inexpensive wall sconces from any hardware or lighting store. The large majority of these sconces hang easily on a nail and plug right into any outlet. Be careful to use no more than seventy-five-watt bulbs on each side to mellow the overhead fluorescent.

Above all, remember my external lighting truths: You *never* have to add fluorescent lights to your incandescent ones. You must *always* add incandescent lighting to your fluorescent. Avoid overlighting that washes away the true color of your makeup. And consider daylight as forever a blessing!

PUTTING ON YOUR DAY FACE

Take out your tool box and open that cosmetic kit. You'll need almost everything to complete a beautiful daytime face. But remember not to overdo the makeup! You have to be understated enough to appear natural in glowing sunshine. Also, your eyes and cheeks should be paler during the day than they are at night.

Establishing a great makeup routine won't take too much practice; however, you can't

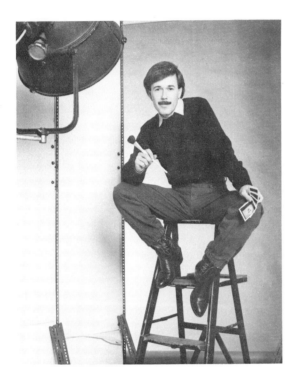

expect to get through your initial makeover without step-by-step instructions. There's an awful lot to learn at first. All the regular application techniques are used in putting on the basic day look. Plus, we each require at least a few of those tricky illusions for fixing minor problems here and there.

So, I've recruited famous makeup artist and hair stylist Jimmy Weis to help me show you the way. I met Jimmy while working on a catalog for a large department store. He immediately homed in on every facial need a fuller-figure woman is concerned about. What else would you expect from a man who has taught beauty around the world for the past thirteen years? Jimmy has also found time to do the makeup and hair for the film *Movieola*, Revlon commercials, and magazines such as *Vogue, Harper's Bazaar,* and *Mademoiselle.*

Now, Jimmy Weis will do a full daytime makeover on me from scratch. As he works, I'll describe how Jimmy does the general application steps. I'll also tell you how he handles my fairly common facial shortcomings. Then, at the end of each step, we'll give you tips on correcting the kinds of imperfections you may be facing.

Eyes first

Many women with average or smaller eyes want big flashing ones. Why not? The eyes are supposed to be the most prominent and expressive part of your face. So, Jimmy naturally starts off by drastically enlarging my puny peepers. You can use the same tricks for opening your eyes.

Doing my eyes first also gives Jimmy the chance to work freely without ruining the foundation. Powders can spill over from my lids. Eyeshadow can get a bit messy. Even black streaks of mascara won't bother a bare face.

TWEEZING

Defining your eyebrows is good preparation for making up your eyes. Eyebrows frame and accentuate the eyes below. The length of your brows effect whether your face is in proportion. And the shape of your eyebrows figure into the tone of your whole look.

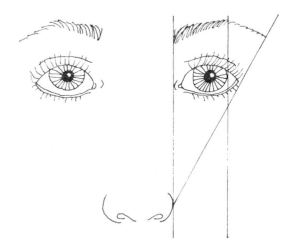

Jimmy first finds the arch of my brows. These are always over the colored part of the eye. Next, he determines the length of my brows by seeing where two sets of imaginary lines intersect my brow lines. The first imaginary line is drawn vertically across the inside corner of my eyelid. Jimmy draws the second one diagonally from the base of my nose to the crown of my head. That's it—the beginning and end of my brows.

Jimmy allows the shape of my brows to follow the brow bones as much as possible. A natural arch is the trend for the eighties. Just look at people like Brooke Shields, Mariel Hemingway, and Jacqueline Bisset. Jimmy then plucks the brows so they appear neat without getting too narrow. Skinny brows on a full face look absolutely silly! The distance between my brows is kept about equal to the width of one of my eyes. After tweezing, Jimmy presses ice cubes to the area to minimize redness or swelling.

Close-set eyes Tweeze brows back to just above the inner corner of the eyes. This puts more light between the eyes.

Wide-set eyes Don't tweeze any hair from

the center of the brows and strengthen inner edges with a brow pencil. Remove a few hairs from outer fringe of brows. Not too much!

Deep-set eyes Pluck your brows thinner to bring more light to the eyes. Please, not too thin!

EYE PENCILING

Before starting to shape my eyes, Jimmy puts two drops of eyeshadow base on my clean eyelids. He blends it in gently to get an even layer over the lid. When you do this step, be careful not to tug at the tissue around the eye. Jimmy also adds a dash of baby powder to the eyelids to set the base. A small sable paintbrush is perfect for this job.

A moment later, Jimmy takes the fat black pencil and draws a line under my lower lashes from the middle to the outer edge. He then uses an 1/8-inch artist's brush to delicately stroke the color into the skin. It appears as a dark-to-medium-gray half shadow after the blending. Jimmy is especially concerned about not creating a corner that would close off my already too-small eyes.

On my upper lashes, Jimmy pencils a line that starts heavier in the outside corners and gets progressively thinner until it ends over the iris. This upper line is also toned down with the 1/8-inch brush. One more narrow stretch of black pencil is applied to the crease of my upper lid and blended.

Close-set eyes Use the black pencil to fill in only the outer third of the lid and "fade" or blend toward the center of the eye. Most emphasis with dark pencil is under the lower lid in extreme outer corner. This appears to lift the whites of the eyes.

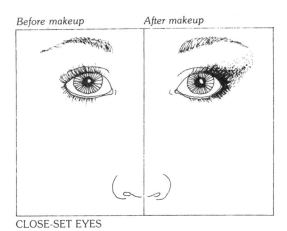

Before makeup   After makeup

CLOSE-SET EYES

Before makeup   After makeup

WIDE-SET EYES

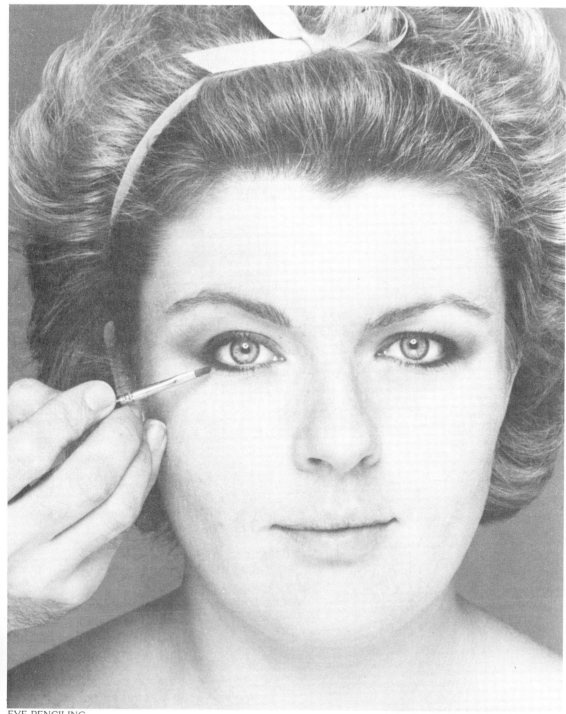

EYE PENCILING

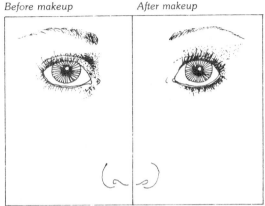

Before makeup   *After makeup*

DEEP-SET EYES

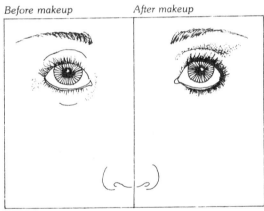

Before makeup   *After makeup*

BULGING EYES

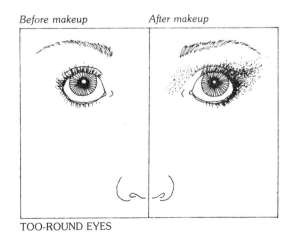

Before makeup   *After makeup*

TOO-ROUND EYES

Wide-set eyes Line eyes evenly all the way around with black pencil.

Deep-set eyes Don't ever use black pencil on your eyes!

Bulging eyes Use a smoky grey pencil around the perimeter of the eyes.

Too-round eyes Pencil shadow only at the ends of the upper and lower lids. Blend it out and upward to create a slant to your eyes.

EYE POWDERING

Powders are used to deflect light and emphasize the hollow of the eye. They make the hollow of the eye stand out or appear to come forward. This opens up the look of the eye. Your eyes seem to grow larger when your eye powder is on just right.

Jimmy first applies the paler eyeshadow powder or highlighter along the length of my upper lid, from my eyelashes to the brow bone. He uses peach shade to complement my hazel eyes. Jimmy prefers to do this with a sponge-tipped applicator, but you can also get by with a powder shadow brush.

The main shadow, plum in my case, is then put on with the small brush over the peach color. It goes into the crease of the lid and spread is from the center of the lid on out. Jimmy then blends it upward to 1/8 inch below the brow line.

He finishes powdering my eyes by dipping the small brush again into the plum shadow and gingerly stroking it under the bottom lid. Jimmy blends the powder in to create a slight shadow beneath the lashes, which makes them appear thicker. This is also a way of emphasizing the perimeter of the eye. But, once

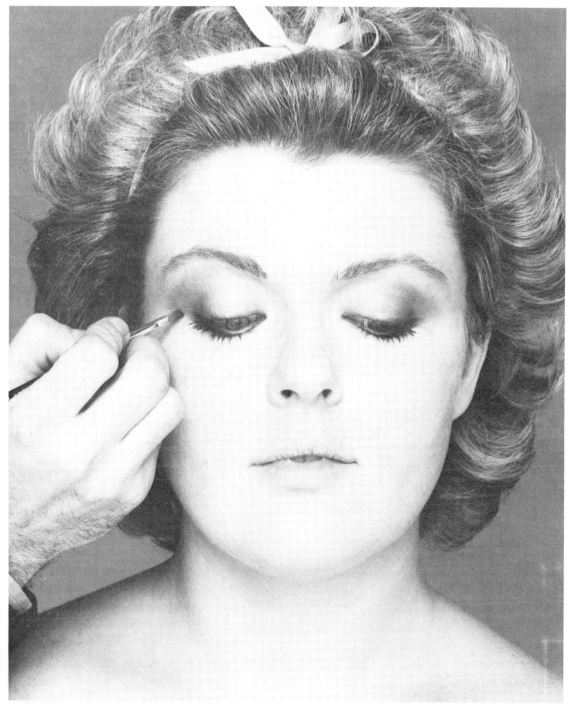

EYE POWDERING (UPPER LID)

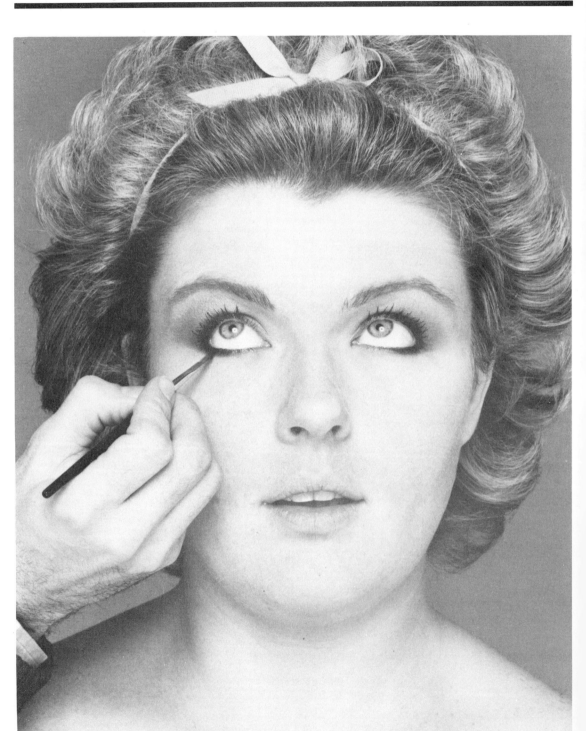

EYE POWDERING (BOTTOM LID)

more, Jimmy avoids closing in my small eyes by keeping clear of the corners.

Close-set eyes Light eyeshadow powder goes on the inside corners of the eyes to widen the look. *No* darker shadow here, ever! Then use medium shadow powder in outer third of upper lid crease and blend it diagonally upward to the brow bone.

Wide-set eyes Light eyeshadow powder goes on the outer corners of the upper lids. Put a smoky, darker powder on the inner corners of the upper lids and blend it to just over the iris so that it mixes with the lighter shade.

Deep-set eyes Hide the darkness by using palest eyeshadow powder over entire lid up to the brow. No shading at all in the crease of the upper lid. This will help bring eye forward too.

Bulging eyes Medium eyeshadow powder goes on the whole upper lid. Blend it both up to 1/8 inch from brow and out toward the temple. This gives your eye a Cleopatra softening effect.

Too-round eyes A medium eyeshadow powder goes on the inner corner of the eyes and is blended toward the center. A slightly darker shadow powder goes from the center of the eyelid out to the temple and up toward the brow bone.

SPARKLING EYES

We decide to take the colorful powders a step further and make my eyes literally sparkle. Jimmy uses an iridescent lavender pencil to catch the highlights of my hazel eyes. You should consult the chart to see what's best for the color of your eyes.

A narrow rim is drawn under the brow arch. Jimmy softens it with an 1/8-inch brush. He also applies the sparkler pencil to the base of the lower lashes and blends.

Close-set eyes Apply sparkler pencil to area under brow arch and out toward the temple.

Wide-set eyes A line of sparkler pencil goes under the brow arch and beneath the outer third of the lower lashes.

Deep-set eyes Use sparkler pencil under the whole arch of brow and under lower lashes for brightening.

Bulging eyes Apply sparkler pencil 1/8-inch below entire brow line.

Too-round eyes Sparkler pencil applied under the arch of the brow and under the outer third of the lower lashes helps.

LOVELY LASHES

My lashes are as straight as an arrow. Too straight! They have to be lifted and curled upward away from my eyes. This gives them a clearer, more appealing configuration. Short, jutting lashes need the same treatment. Eyelash curlers provide that glamorous little twist.

Jimmy slips my top lashes halfway into the curler, squeezes it easily together for a few seconds and releases. Too tight a grasp tends to leave a crease or ninety-degree angle in your lashes. He's also careful not to place the curler too close to the rim of the lid. The last thing I want is the pain of lashes being pulled out— Ouch!

After the lashes are curled, the mascara goes on. Jimmy covers only the outer portions of my upper lashes. Then he separates any clumps with a brow brush.

Close-set eyes Only put mascara on the outer bottom and top lashes.

Wide-set eyes Apply mascara evenly to all lashes.

Deep-set eyes Lots of mascara on lower and upper lashes.

Bulging eyes Put mascara on just the outer lashes.

Too-round eyes Mascara on the outer lashes takes away roundness.

CLEANING UP

All that's left is the cleaning job, which gets my face ready for the contouring ahead. Jimmy dips a Q-tip into eye-makeup remover and meticulously wipes away excess powders. He makes certain not to touch the shadows on my lids or the other areas just done up. I notice that Jimmy always wipes in an upward swing from the side of the nose to the temple. Finally, Jimmy blends in any still-harsh powder lines and blots excess remover with a tissue.

Pre-foundation touch-ups

Jimmy dabs a small amount of glycerine under my eyes, around the bottom of my nose, and on the edges of my mouth—you know, that area where nasty smile lines grow. All of these spots lack oil glands and are wrinkle prone. The glycerine holds in the moisture that's naturally there, which gives the skin a dewy look. Moisturizing also prevents foundation and powder from caking into crevices.

By the way, this is where Jimmy decides to enrich my pale skin with some violet *color corrector*. He dots just a small amount to my

face and works it in. Check the color-corrector chart (page 43) to see what color might do you some good.

Contouring and highlighting illusions

Contouring is the use of a darker foundation to diminish areas that are too wide. Highlighting is the use of a very light foundation or opaque concealer to bring out areas that are too small. By combining them skillfully, you can change the shape of your face, eliminate double chins, or remodel the line of your nose. Jimmy does all those things to make my face beautiful.

FACE SHAPING

My face is a combination heart and square shape, but for the sake of contouring, it's treated like a heart. After all, the top of my head is much broader than the bottom. Our aim is, of course, to create the impression of an oval-shaped face. Always strive for the ultimate oval.

Jimmy applies a medium shade of foundation first to my temples and the sides of my forehead. He dots it on with his fingers and blends it in well toward the hairline. Overdoing the contouring gives your skin a muddy, dirty look. Heavier contouring is only for dim lights or night maneuvers. Remember to use the arch of your eyebrow as a guideline for the inner edge of the contouring.

Now Jimmy dabs highlighter to my chin and the outer edges of each side of my chin. Again the lighter foundation is spread only as far as an imaginary line dropped vertically from the arch of my eyebrows. We've created the illusion of an evenly proportioned

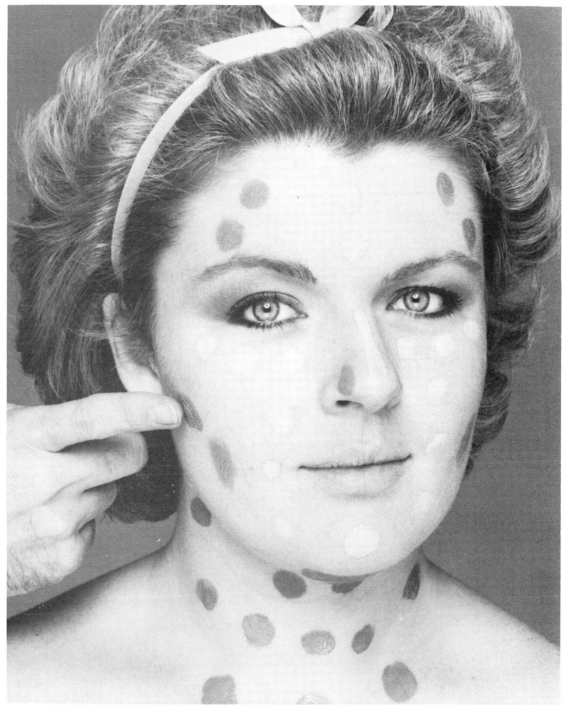

CONTOURING AND HIGHLIGHTING ILLUSIONS

Before makeup   After makeup

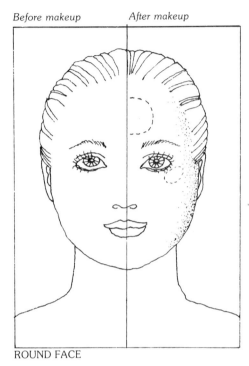

ROUND FACE

Before makeup   After makeup

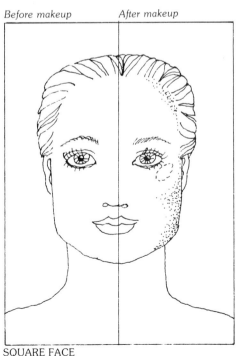

SQUARE FACE

forehead and chin. All light seems to be concentrated in the center of my face and away from the imperfections we want to hide.

All face shapes discussed in Chapter 3 can be contoured into a facsimile of the ultimate oval. Of course, the few fuller-figure women with oval faces can just quit while they're ahead. For the rest of you it will take a few well-directed dots. Find your face shape and follow these simple tips.

Round faces Dot darker foundation on either side of your face in the shape of a crescent that runs from the hairline to the sides of the jaw. Blend it into a shadow that makes your face look longer and thinner. Speckle highlighter in the center of your forehead and under your eyes (just above the cheekbones). Again, blend well.

Square faces Put darker foundation at all four corners of your square face (the right angles of each side of the forehead and jawline). This softens the angles when they're blended gently. Place a little additional contour below the cheekbones and spread softly toward the ears. This creates a hollow, which helps ovalize your square. Dot highlight above your cheekbones to help make the eyes stand out.

Diamond faces Poke some darker foundation on the temples where the face is too broad. This narrows your face when blended. Use highlighter on the center of your forehead and on the jawline to broaden them. It will add up to an oval.

Triangular faces Darker foundation is dotted along your jawline to soften the corners at the bottom of the triangle. Blend smoothly. Put a drop of contour on the cheekbones and

Before makeup   *After makeup*

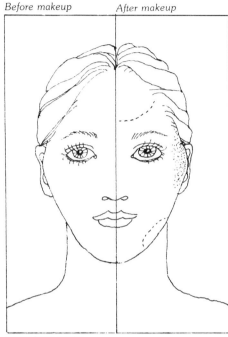

DIAMOND FACE

Before makeup   *After makeup*

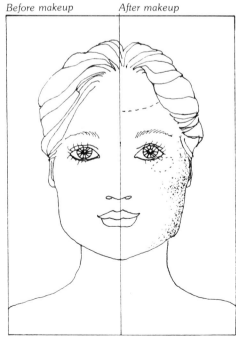

TRIANGULAR FACE

just below them to emphasize the area. Highlight the forehead to make it appear broader. A little highlighter can also go under the eyes to bring them out.

DARKENING DOUBLE CHINS

Extra attention is given to hiding my double chin. I know some of you could use the same solution. Jimmy applies the darker foundation to the area that hangs. He then dots opaque concealer on either side and below the double chin and is careful to blend outward. This draws attention to my face and away from the spare chin.

FIXING THE NOSE

Before moving on, Jimmy does a little painless cosmetic surgery on my *too-wide nose*. First, he finds how wide my nose should be by drawing two imaginary vertical lines through the center of my nostrils toward the brows. Then, he removes the surplus on either side by dotting on the contour to cover it all up. A thin line of highlighter is drawn down the middle of my nose to draw attention away from the sides.

A *thin nose* would be corrected by putting highlighter on the sides. *Long noses* are shortened by contouring the tip and underside of the nostrils. A *hook nose* is leveled by darkening the prominent bone. A *crooked nose* is centered by darkening the bent side and highlighting the other side.

NARROWING THE NECK

Slenderizing your face and facial features is not enough. Jimmy completes the contouring job by working wonders on my *short, thick*

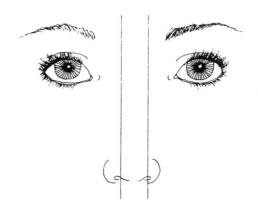

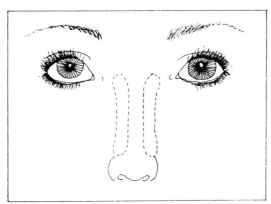

THIN NOSE

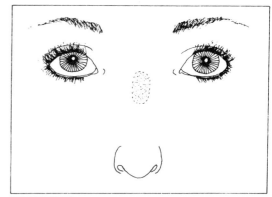

HOOK NOSE

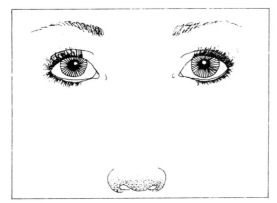

LONG NOSE

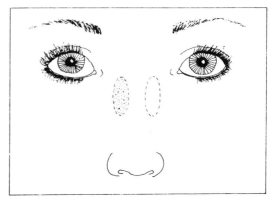

CROOKED NOSE

neck. He applies the darker coloring to my neck in the shape of a man's collar and tie. That means shading an inverted triangle on either side of my neck and another right down the middle. Keep the shaded areas narrow and blend them in.

Long, thick necks can also be thinned with some contouring. Apply darker foundation in the shape of a high, narrow Victorian collar. Shading goes from just below the ears to the collarbones. Here the front of the neck is untouched.

Laying the overall foundation

Contouring and highlighting represents only two-thirds of the total foundation. Overall foundation provides the background and texture for your facial illusions, but there are other steps necessary for finishing off your final layer of foundation in the proper fashion. Jimmy does them on me in the following order.

1 He applies *yellow concealer* to my chin to cover a blemish and to my cheek to hide enlarged capillaries. When he smoothes the concealer in it helps even my skin tone.

2 Jimmy then dots *basic or overall foundation* on my forehead, nose, cheeks, lips, chin, and neck. The light shade—appropriate for my pale skin—is blended in gently with his fingertips. Check the foundation color chart (page 44) for your correct shade.

3 After all the foundation is on, Jimmy *sponges off* the excess. He blends gently with the sponge in an upward motion. Pressing too hard could smear the contour. When he finishes, my complexion has a creamy look.

4 *Translucent powder* is generously applied with

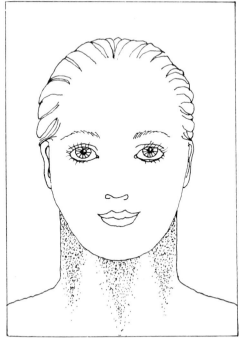

SHORT, THICK NECK

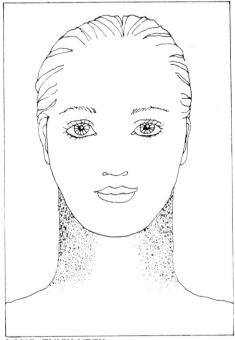

LONG, THICK NECK

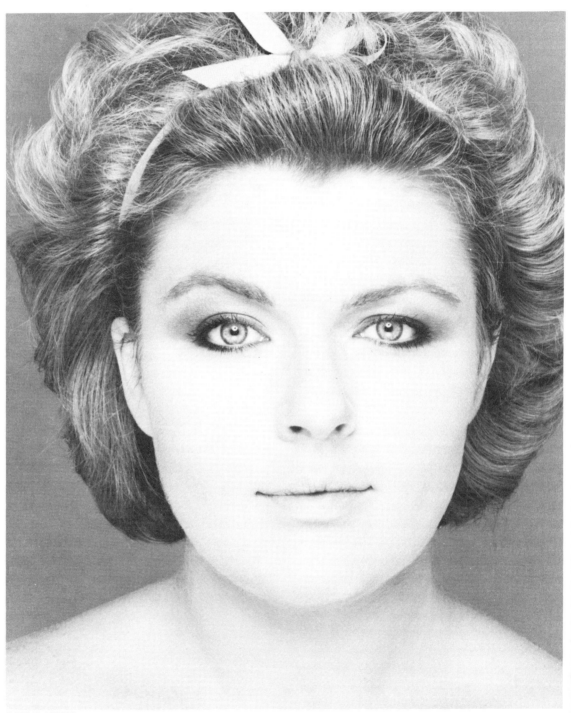

FOUNDATION

a large powder brush to any spot previously covered by foundation. The other large powder brush then sweeps the powder away from the center of the face. This removes excess powder and starts setting my makeup. (Older women with wrinkled skin should use very little powder, since excess powder will settle in and accentuate wrinkles.) Jimmy also puts an ice cube in a plastic bag and presses it against my face to promote further setting.

A youthful blush

Blushers are put on lightly to give your cheeks a healthy and very natural glow. This is not the kind of coloring you smear all over your face. Jimmy defines the area to be blushed by drawing one imaginary line from the outer corner of my mouth to the outer corner of my eye. A second imaginary border is sketched from the same eye corner to where my ear begins. All blushing is done between these two lines.

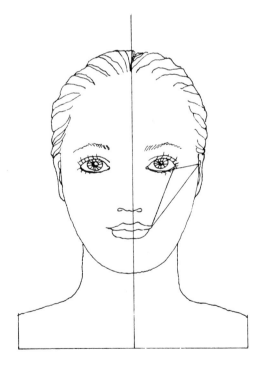

Jimmy decides to use three shades of blush on my face, but you can get away with just the first two. The lightest shade or *main blush* goes on before the others. In my case, Jimmy solidly brushes on a mauve blush over my cheekbones. He brushes it in an outward direction and is careful to avoid streaks or striping.

A pink *accent blusher* is added just below my cheekbones for extra depth. Check the color chart (page 44) to see which shades of blush are right for you.

Here Jimmy brings in a third *blending blusher*. He brushes the blending color (again pink) around the edges of the blush area. This

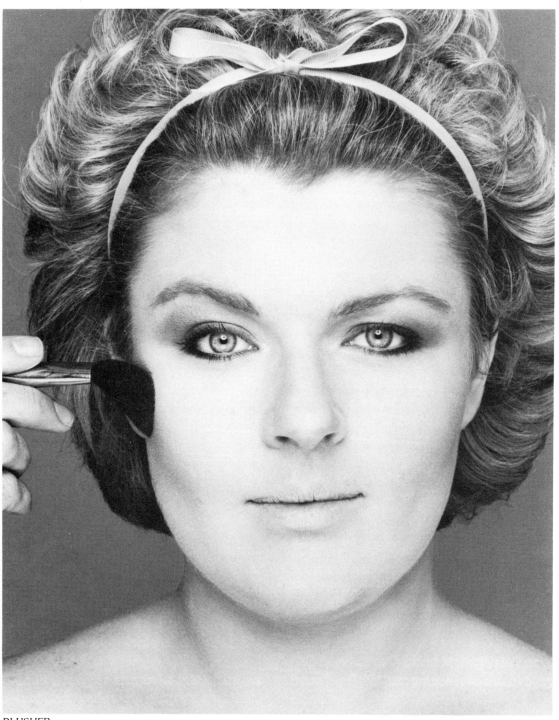

BLUSHER

makes the blush soften gradually into the rest of my face and gives a more natural appearance.

Brow penciling

Surprise! Just before doing my lips Jimmy takes an unexpected detour back to my eyebrows. It's always smart to pencil in your brows after you see the general color and contour of your face. The brows should be only a hint of color framing the eyes. Never make your eyebrows so overpowering that people see them before noticing the eyes or anything else. Joan Crawford was infamous for that makeup mistake.

Jimmy uses a medium shade to fill in gaps in my dark brows. Always use a pencil one shade lighter than your eyebrows. The brows must be subtle, but uniform. Penciling also helps to etch more precisely the line of the brow.

Luscious lips

Your lips go on last. But never allow them to be the least important part of your makeup. The lips should be expressive, sensual, moist, and always in proportion to your face.

My lips happen to be distinctly uneven. I have a narrow upper lip and an overly full lower lip. Jimmy uses a *flesh-colored lip pencil* to draw a lip line that corrects my imbalance. He sketches the line of my lower lip inside the natural edge. My upper lip is penciled along the natural border. After the line is complete, a Q-tip is used to gently blend the penciling into a faint shadow around the perimeter of my mouth.

Jimmy adds to the illusion by using a clear red *lipstick* on my lower lip and a slightly lighter shade on my upper lip. The difference in color makes my lips seem more balanced. A lipstick brush makes the application smoother. My pencil border will also prevent the lipstick from "bleeding" onto the skin around my mouth.

No matter how great my lips turn out, touch-ups will be needed throughout the day. Be sure to carry your lipstick and lipstick brush with you. Keep your lips luscious.

OTHER KINDS OF LIP LAMENTS

Here's a few hot tips to use as a smoke screen to hide other lip problems.

Too-full lips Draw a narrow lip inside the natural borders of both your top and bottom lips. This will make them look thinner when filled in. Don't use lip gloss! It will only make your already thick lips look fuller.

Narrow lips Pencil an outline beyond the natural edges of your lips. This will make your mouth appear fuller. Don't overdo it! Just a fraction of an inch makes a big difference. Fill in your lips with a light shade of lipstick. Remember, light stands out and dark recedes. Finish the effect off with some gloss in the center of your lips. The gloss accentuates the middle of the mouth and adds to the illusion of fullness.

YOUR FIVE-MINUTE EMERGENCY MAKEOVER

You've just completed the full, most fantastic daytime face imaginable. I know it took quite a while to get it right the first time out. Practice just a little and you'll be simply gorgeous

TOO-FULL LIPS

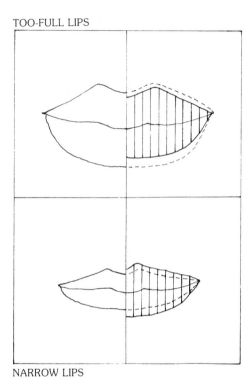

NARROW LIPS

in fifteen to twenty minutes. Eventually, you'll be creating beautiful illusions in your sleep.

Most women find the basic day face easy enough to fit into their daily schedule. Get up, make up, breakfast, run for the 8-o'clock express. However, there are times when you're running late or only want to drop down to the store on a sleepy Sunday. Do you go out bare faced or spend twenty minutes you don't have making up?

Neither! This is the time to leap into your bathroom for the amazing *five-minute emergency face*—faster than a speeding bullet and more attractive than no makeup at all. It'll give you a super lift in time of crisis. Here's how you do it.

1 Forget the tweezing and eyebrow pencil altogether.

2 Quickly line your eyes with eyeshadow pencil as suggested in the regular section on eyeshadow penciling. Smudge with a stroke or two.

3 Skip the three layers of blusher. Use a light color wash in the same area. *Don't* overdo to compensate.

4 Abandon any ideas about contouring or highlighting. Even overall foundation takes too much time to apply.

5 Just lightly tint your lips with lip gloss, top and bottom. This is no time to worry about balanced lips.

Finished in five minutes or less. Admittedly, not your captivating, slimmer-than-the-real-you face. But, it's a pretty-enough look to make even the grocer take notice.

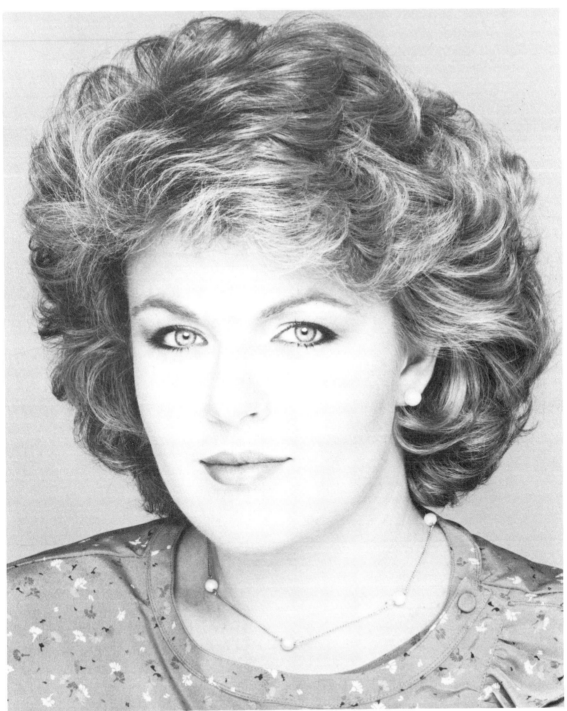

FINISHED DAY FACE

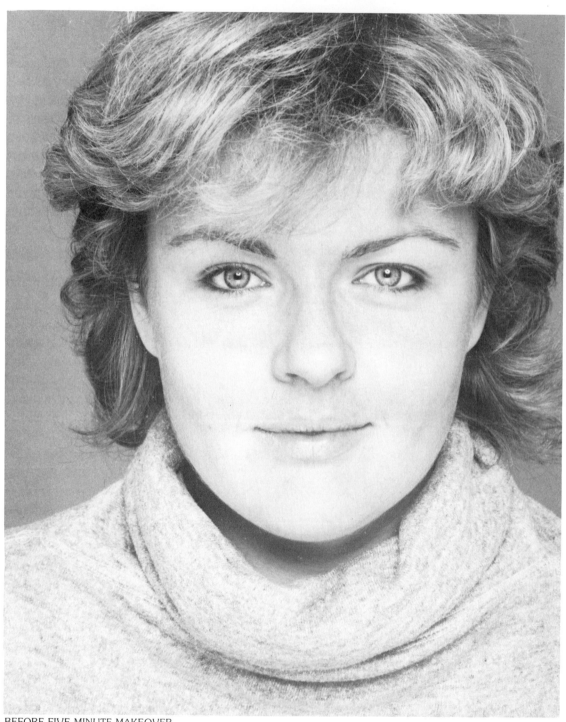

BEFORE FIVE-MINUTE MAKEOVER

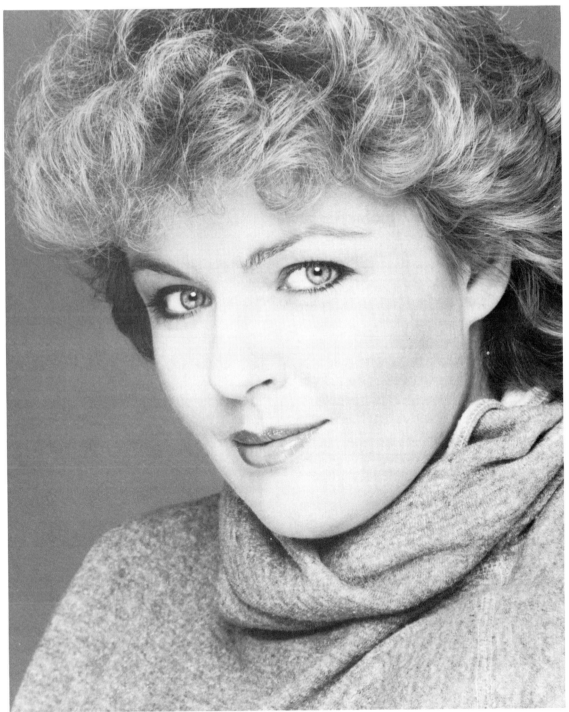

AFTER FIVE-MINUTE MAKEOVER

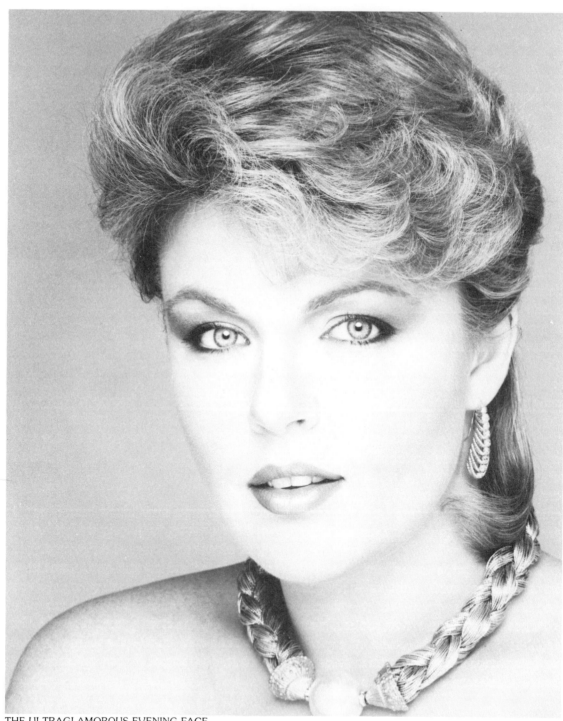

THE ULTRAGLAMOROUS EVENING FACE

THE ULTRAGLAMOROUS EVENING FACE

Touching up your day face can get you through an after-work drink or a night at the neighborhood movie theater. However, those extra-special nights out on the town require something a bit more striking. Let's really get dramatic! It only takes a few more minutes to do than the basic day face.

In fact, let's start the fabulous evening look where the daytime makeup leaves off. I'll only be giving you the steps that embellish the already done day face. Jimmy will do his applications in the same order as before— beginning with my eyes—so there's no chance for confusion. Remember to refer back to the notes on your particluar face shape and other special features. Okay, here's the stunning evening additions.

Evening eyes

Jimmy decides to add some black pencil to the outside corners of my eyes. They appear even bigger than before, and the whites gleam. Black pencil also redefines the rim of my eyes. They're darker all the way around, but the inside corners are still left open. A brush is used to blend it.

My eyelids are now dressed up with some pearlized powders. These match the color of the powders I'm already wearing. Jimmy wants to make my lids shimmer without turning them into a kaleidoscope. Another pale powder is brushed over the brow bone to extend the shimmer.Sparkler is penciled under the brow arch and along the base of my lower lashes. Everything is blended gently.

Twinkle, twinkle, pretty eyes! All systems are go. But Jimmy stops long enough to brush away excess powder and clean up under my eyes.

Face glitter

You've already done enough contouring and highlighting for the day face. But you can wake up your foundation with some sparkly translucent powder. It comes loose and spreads on thick. If you prefer a matte finish, stick to your regular day powder.

Jimmy further electrifies my face with an extra coat of blushers. Night's dim lights allow for a heavier hand with colors. But the secret is to keep on blending, blending, blending. Of course, this evening blush comes with lustrous sparkles of its own.

Flashy brows

Subdued brows can brighten up in the gloom of night. Jimmy fills in my dark eyebrows with gold-beige pencil, an ideal evening shade for most women. He uses a brow brush to blend it into the skin. Then, a few swipes of the brush fluffs the brows into flashy streaks over my eyes.

Sultry lips

In the evening my lips get a brighter and darker color lipstick. Jimmy puts the darker color everywhere, except in the center of my lower lip. Here a lighter shade creates a sexy "pout." Lip gloss or shiner on that same center spot adds a "come-hither" sparkle.

The rest is fate, attitude, and the glint of the moonlight.

CHAPTER FIVE

FACE SAVERS

After making up, I feel especially pretty, and get a kick from just looking in the mirror. But don't think of cosmetics as the whole beauty treatment for your face. Not by a long shot! The crucial routines first begin when your colorful powders, creams, and lipsticks come off.

Taking care of your facial skin is the key to lasting beauty. What's the sense of painting a lovely portrait on a flaky, dirty, or oily canvas? Our problem is that most of us don't know enough about keeping a healthy complexion. We believe every product hype or mythical remedy.

The majority of women I speak to aren't even sure what kind of skin they have. Wondering what type you are? There's an easy way to find out. I'll also give you some tips on cleaning, toning, moisturizing, and protecting your face from the elements. Then after consulting Dr. Ira Gouterman, chief of dermatology at St. Michael's Medical Center, Newark, New Jersey, we are able to pose some cures for annoying complexion disorders such as acne and enlarged capillaries. As an added incentive, at the end of the chapter, there is a list of homemade facial masks guaranteed to leave you tingling from the neck up.

SKIN TYPES

The process for determining your skin type takes very little effort, yet it does call for a bit of wait-and-see time. So try to pick a long, lazy morning for doing the following steps. In fact, you can even get up early and then pop back to sleep for a while.

Start by washing your face with pure soap and water. Please, don't add any fancy supplements today. Then gently pat yourself dry with a soft towel. We don't want to irritate anything. Now, just let your face breathe for two or three hours.

The waiting period gives your skin time to secrete the fluids it naturally produces. Then, when you study your face in the makeup mirror, the reflection will show what your skin is really like. For instance, an overall shine means you have *oily skin*. A flaky face without any shine suggests a *dry skin* type. However, like most fuller-figure women, you'll probably see a shiny T stretching across your forehead and down along your nose and chin.

This T brands you as having a *combination* oily-down-the-middle-and-dry-on-the-sides complexion. It's not as ominous as it sounds. All three categories require some special considerations. But with smart skin-care routines anybody can have a uniformly smooth, clear face. Here are some specific methods for making the most of your skin type.

SOFT-SOAPING YOUR FACE

Each kind of skin has to be washed a different way. Still, there are some general cleaning rules that apply to everybody. First of all, reach for the old-fashioned bar of soap. It's easily the most *effective* agent for removing makeup or the accumulated grime of the day. But don't lather up just any old soap. Many brands on the market tend to be too alkaline

and irritating. Read the ingredients on the wrapper carefully before purchase.

Never rub a deodorant soap on your sensitive facial skin. Those coarse perfumes are meant for the body only. Likewise, avoid using fad cleaners such as mayonnaise. I know it's being recommended by others in the beauty field, but, most mayonnaises contain preservatives, which can cause irritations. If you want to try some helpful facial recipes, I'll give you a kitchenful later on.

Washcloths can also be more trouble than they're worth. It's unhealthy to pull the same worn rag across your face over and over again. Bacteria breeds in a moist place quicker than you think. So, either go for a fresh washcloth *every* time or use your hands, like I do.

Let your fingers massage your skin in an upward, circular motion as you wash. Be careful not to tug at the tissue around your eyes. I play it safe by using a cotton ball and light mineral oil to take off any stubborn eye makeup. Don't *scrub* any part of your face. That's strictly for floors and potatoes.

Washing your skin type

Oily skin is not an open invitation to wash, wash, wash. Overwashing your face only encourages the skin to produce more natural oils. Eventually your skin will be manufacturing a lot more oil than your're soaking away. But moderate washing is still necessary.

In addition to soap and water, your cleansing routine should include a fat-free substance for removing excess oil. Cetaphil is a liquid cleanser that gets rid of accumulated oils without totally stripping your skin. High-alkaline soaps remove all oils and leave your face too dry and scaly.

Dry skin should also be washed only a couple of times a day. Make sure you use a low-alkaline soap that contains cold cream. Dove is the most popular of these soaps. Cold-cream soaps clean the skin while forming a thin layer of moisture on the surface. This should help prevent flaking.

Combination skin is first cleansed all over with a low-alkaline soap and water. Then the oily T gets an extra dose of skin toner, and the dry outer areas receive a liberal amount of moisturizer.

Toner treats and taboos

Toners can be a blessing or a curse. You usually apply them after washing your face. They remove any traces of soap from your skin and help to close your pores. A good toner even gives a special freshness to your complexion. But an astringent can do some serious damage to your skin.

Astringents are toners with a high alcohol content. Most women with dry skin know enough to stay away from the severe drying power of alcohol products. Unfortunately though, there's a myth about astringents being the perfect remedy for oily skin. That's a dangerous misconception! Astringents can overstrip the most oily face and trigger a deluge of oil to take its place. Obviously a vicious cycle.

Nonalcoholic toners, however, should be embraced by large women. They pamper our skin in warm or dry climates. When the toner is refrigerated, it perks up your face and makes it tingle to the touch. If the toner stings, you should either dilute it or return it to the store.

Harper's toner recipes

One way to get around overly strong store-bought toners is to whip up a batch of your own. I regularly make up *three* different kinds for myself. Each one has a light touch that does the trick just fine.

☐ Mix 1 part apple-cider vinegar to 7 parts of either tap or bottled water. Shake well.

☐ Put ½ teaspoon of mint extract into 2 cups of water. Mix it with vigor.

☐ Add 1 part witch hazel (15 percent alcohol) to 4 parts water. Women with oily skin will thrive on the low alcohol content, but this is *not* for women with dry skin.

Sealing in moisture

Moisturizers come in many different forms. I've seen lotions, creams (day and night), sprays, and everything in between. Yet not one of these actually restores moisture to the skin. It just doesn't work that way.

Moisturizers are sealants more than anything else. Fluids are already in the skin even when it appears dry. What we're hoping to do is prevent moisture from being stolen by our environment. As a result, the best moisturizer for the top layer of skin is something like petroleum jelly. But who wants to walk around with that smeared of her face?

Well, you don't have to show the world a greasy visage. If you have exceptionally dry skin—often a side effect of aging—do your moisturizing at night after washing off the makeup. A hot bath sets up your face very well. Then put on a thin layer of Eucerin or petroleum jelly. Don't use very heavy creams that can clog your pores and result in skin eruptions.

During the day you can follow the advice I give in Chapter 4 about glycerine, which is great for moisturizing the areas around the eyes, nostrils and mouth. Remember, these areas have no oil glands, so apply the glycerine before daytime cosmetics.

In reading the ingredients found in most moisturizers, you'll see that water heads the list. Yes, the very liquid we accused of robbing oils from your skin. However, in this instance it works to your advantage. As the water evaporates it helps to draw the face-smoothing elements—glycerine, lanolin, or mineral oil—into your skin. These act as protectors that seal the skin without smothering it.

Instead of worrying about what's in or not in a brand-name moisturizer, simply make your own. I've left lanolin out of my concoction because it can aggravate acne-prone skin. But the ingredients included are sufficent to do the job. This is my mild, everyday moisturizer. Mix it up well like a long, cool drink.

one part glycerine and rose water
one part mineral oil
two parts water

THE RULES OF WRINKLING

Everybody wrinkles somewhat as they get older. That's absolutely unavoidable. However, fuller-figure women normally have much less of a problem with wrinkles because our fat tends to bolster the facial skin and keep it from sagging. It's only when we go through very rapid weight loss that our skin loses some of its elasticity.

Isometric exercises, can minimize wrinkling due to weight loss. But they can't reverse a severe sagging problem. Many "wrinkle creams" temporarily remove wrinkles by irritating the skin so that it swells up. This stretches the wrinkles out, and you appear to look smoother. Of course, once the swelling disappears, your old wrinkles return.

According to Dr. Gouterman, expensive collagen products don't do the trick either. Collagen is the substance that makes up the bottom layer of your skin. The sales pitches suggest that if you put a collagen product on your face it will remove wrinkles by replenishing the natural composition of your skin. "It's like putting a hunk of steak in a spaghetti colander," says Gouterman, "and expecting it to pass through to the other side."

There is nothing capable of curing your wrinkles once they're ingrained on your face. Damage done by aging and sun exposure, the reasons for ninety-five percent of our wrinkles, is permanent. All we can do is start to protect ourselves against wrinkling as early as possible. Those of you who are between the ages of fifteen and twenty-eight can do a lot to keep your skin youthful. Older women must work to slow down any further wrinkling.

Saving your face
FROM THE ELEMENTS

It doesn't matter if it's hot, cold, wet, or dry. Each kind of climate presents a real threat to your face. Exposure to the elements can cause blotching, blisters, chafing, and acne. I know you can't hide your face under the blankets, but you can think about your skin before stepping out the front door.

Sunburn is the devil of all weather worries. A bright day entices you to frolic on the beach and stare up at the sun. But take some precautions first. For starters, don't use soap with hexachlorophene during the summer; it may photosensitize your face and make you prone to developing nasty red blisters.

Sun-blocking products should be worn religiously at the beach. Where is it written that we must tan immediately—or at all? I'm not allowed to tan during part of the summer when I have to shoot winter catalogs. And I still manage to enjoy myself.

On goes a stylish, wide-brimmed hat to shade my face. My lips and eyes sport a little cosmetic color. A fetching swimsuit lifts my spirits. You'd be surprised how many men overlook my lack of reddish-tan.

By the way, you don't have to be down at the shore to face the ravages of sunburn. Those of you living in high altitudes should be aware that you're exposed to even more of the sun's ultraviolet rays. Skiers also get extra doses of sun reflecting off the snow. Use sunscreens on your face and lip balms on your mouth. Some skiers even resort to a little petroleum jelly for their cheeks and nose.

Tropical humidity is especially rough on fuller-figure women. Our additional weight causes the sebaceous glands to produce more oils. Here heavy moisturizers and thick sunscreens can badly clog pores when we perspire. The key is to avoid the midday sun and use light moisturizers, like glycerine and rose water. What's more, stay out of saunas and steam rooms if you want to keep your face clear.

Extreme temperatures, both the *cold* northern winters and the *arid* desert seasons, promote severe dryness. Try not to expose your face to water more than twice a day. When you do wash, the water should be lukewarm —never scalding hot. In the morning and evening put on a thin layer of petroleum jelly (or my moisturizer, page 73) to keep your skin from getting flaky or itchy.

Healing complexion ills

Our faces are particularly susceptible to a few embarrassing skin disorders, the kinds of ailments that hurt your ego more than your overall health. But why wait until you have the problem to seek a solution. Here's what you should look out for and what to do when you find it.

Enlarged capillaries are common in overweight women. Our fuller faces need a denser network of capillaries to keep the fatty tissue thriving. Normally, these tiny blood vessels swell up and shrink hundreds of times a day. But a problem occurs when things in our diet overstimulate the capillaries. They just continue to grow bigger and bigger. Finally, when they do shrink back, it's to a somewhat enlarged size.

The bulging red marks on your face will usually disappear if you follow some sound advice. Dr. Gouterman suggests cutting down on caffeine and alcohol. He believes that both chemicals cause the capillaries to expand. Favorites like cola, coffee, chocolate, spicy foods, and wine can also do damage.

He also points out that heat can also enlarge blood vessels. The doctor warns against holding a hot cup of tea up to your face. Saunas and steam baths are obviously out. Even hot showers should be cooled down until the vessels contract. In extreme cases a dermatologist can dissolve enlarged capillaries via a process called electrodesiccation.

Acne roseacea, or "adult acne," is another facial skin disorder that tends to plague large women. This looks like teenage acne at a glance, but closer inspection shows a combination of four symptoms. One is a general redness of the face. The second is enlarged capillaries. Little angry pustules are the third sign. And rhinophyma, a rare bulbous enlargement of the nose (associated with W. C. Fields), is the unique fourth symptom.

Adult acne is treated in much the same way you would combat enlarged capillaries. Avoid all the caffeine and alcohol aggravators. Skip the heat-producing situations. Get a dermatologist to examine any extreme outbreaks.

Teenage acne, unlike adult acne, has nothing to do with being heavy. It's a universal skin problem that's simply part of the natural maturation of your oil glands and hormones. Some young women have worse trouble with acne because their glands are more sensitive to the hormones. Don't despair! Time and some intelligent care will heal most wounds.

The best over-the-counter medicine is benzoyl peroxide. Use a cotton ball to apply it in the evening after cleansing your face. Don't expect to dab some on once or twice a week and still see favorable results. It must be a nightly routine. Brand-name acne products cost more than the generic brands. So, check the labels on both before you buy. If you get the generic product, you might wind up with the same mixture for a lot less money.

HOMEMADE FACIAL MASKS

Everything we've discussed up to now fits into a basic face-saving routine. These are things you must do to protect your skin. But once you've done all the basics it's time to pamper yourself with some good-feeling, healthy extras. Facial masks will goose up the skin's circulation, remove flaky skin cells, unclog stubborn pores, and generally add zest to your complexion.

No, I'm not sending you to an expensive spa or salon. Each one of my facial masks can be cooked up for pennies apiece in the privacy of your kitchen. Choose the ones that fit your needs. But if you want to try them all, then stick to this order:

1. A mask of steam

Steaming your face is a great way to open up pores for further cleaning. However, women who are bothered by enlarged capillaries should skip it. This is merely an introductory mask designed to prepare your skin and mellow you out.

I begin by boiling three to four quarts of water in a large, twin-handled pot. After removing it from the stove, I put two tea-spoons of fragrant chamomile tea into the water. Then I sit down on a chair beside the open pot. A large towel is used to enclose my face and head over the pot.

Ah-h-h, the steam rises up and seeps into my pores. I'm lulled by the heat, but remember to stay at least a few inches away. For five to ten minutes I remain hunched over with the towel in place. Now I'm ready for the next step.

2. Yogurt and cornmeal scrub

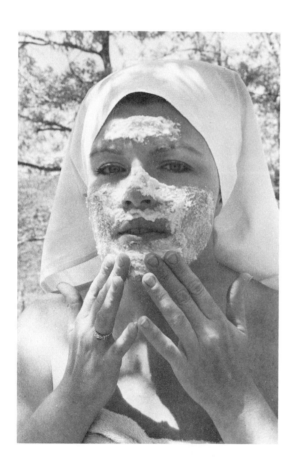

This tasty mask is used as a skin slougher for those who want to shed dead cells. It gives the vibrant layers of your face a chance to breathe. Here's the simple recipe.

Mix three tablespoons of yogurt and one tablespoon of coarse cornmeal together to form a paste. I'm always careful to massage it into my skin gently. I concentrate on covering my T zone. If you don't have a combination complexion, then work the paste all over your face. Every skin type should make a point of covering the neck and chin area, too.

The massaging goes on for about five minutes. If you do not have cornmeal, substitute fine salt or pulverized almonds. At the end, rinse your face with tepid water first, then splash on cold water to close the pores.

3. Dried-egg mask

After sloughing you need a mask to tighten or tone your skin. Walking around with egg on your face is my way of doing it. Sounds silly, but believe me, it works.

Take an egg white and whip it up with a wire wisk. (It's a good exercise for your upper arms.) Then slather the frothy egg on your face. Avoid the area right around your eyes. I keep the egg on my face for about ten to fifteen minutes—or until it's dry. A cool-water rinse follows.

Your skin will feel incredibly smooth and there will be a taut, youthful tone to your face. I'm always surprised at how many people notice the difference.

4. Eye-opening masks

The last kind of facial mask is used to open your eyes after a long sleep. When you doze, water settles into the face, causing puffiness around the eyes. Anything that's cool will bring the swelling down.

If you're feeling lazy, there is a gel mask that you can buy. Just pop it into the refrigerator to chill and then put it on. Wearing it for five minutes in bed before facing the world should be enough. These masks are also great for tired eyes after a long day. It will wake you up for the evening ahead.

I prefer to use some handy fruit or vegetable to soothe my puffy eyes. I take two round slices of chilled cucumber, potato, or apple and place them on my eyes. Then I take five minutes in the soft comfort of my bedroom. When I get up the puffiness is gone. Sometimes, saving your face is so easy you can do it in your sleep.

CHAPTER SIX

HAIR CHANGES

In a decade of modeling, I've had to constantly attack my hair to come up with the right look. Primarily my hair had to fit in with the shape of my face and figure. But I also wanted it to reflect my attitude, age, and the fashionable fads of the times. So I've learned to think of my hair as a personal, ever-changing asset, rather than something to sweep up under a hat.

When I started to get bookings in June of 1972, my then-long hair was streaked blond, with a part down the middle, and soft, flowing strands framing my face. I felt young, attractive, and glad to be out of the binge doldrums. My cascading hairstyle was a way of saying, "I'm free and full of confidence."

By 1974, my modeling identity was secure enough for me to try a less theatrical cut. I opted for a neater, medium length that offered boundless versatility and a touch more sophistication. A couple of years after that, my blond streaks faded into a mellower shade to match what was "in." Currently, my hair is on the short side and naturally wavy, for the active eighties. Like any busy woman, I need a cut that falls into place after jogging, swimming, or a hard day's work. And this hairstyle can easily be modified for an evening of dining and dancing.

Your daily bread might not depend on fitting into the editorial angles of various ads or staying one step in front of the latest hair craze. But occasionally you should try a new style just to keep up with the changes in your

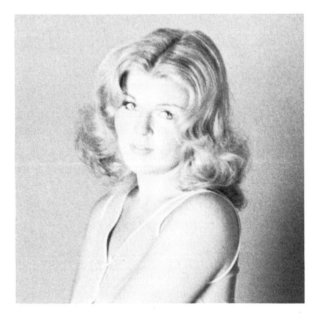

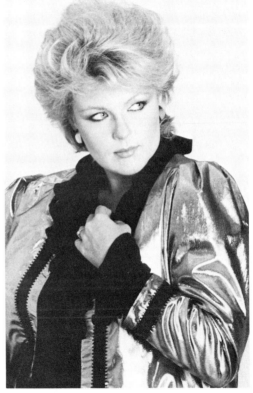

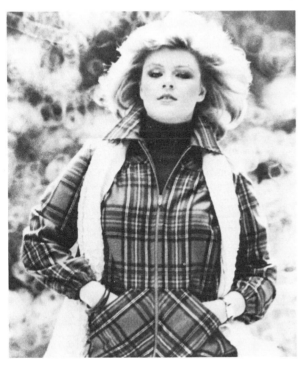

appearance and life-style. Life, looks, and a woman who wants to be beautiful can't stand still! The key is to know how to figure out what suits you at the moment.

You can begin searching for the right hairstyle by giving up the old myth about *long hair* being the beauty cure-all. It barely worked for me years ago, in spite of my height and well-conditioned hair. The truth is most fuller-figure women come off heavier, not sexier, when their tresses dangle to the shoulders or below. A viewer's eyes are drawn to where your hair stops. If your hair intermingles with your body, your size gets all the attention and that pretty face is overlooked. What's more, fine or wispy hair seems even thinner once it grows past the base of your neck.

As a rule, large women should avoid extremes. Mounds of hair piled on the top of the head make us appear bulkier; scalp-hugging cuts shrink the head too much in relation to the body. My philosophy is to use hair as a tool for putting things in proportion and for helping to ovalize the face. Inevitably, almost *everything* about being a Big Beauty comes back to these two points.

By now you should sense that flipsy-dipsy-swirly hairdos are out. Fancy creations flying off every which way are rarely flattering to a large woman. With the assistance of Artistic Director Kim Lepine of New York's sensational La Coupe Salon, I'll guide you instead to simpler styles. These generally come out prettier and are easier to maintain. Then I'll show you how to put body in your hair and how to keep each strand continually healthy. For a finale, La Coupe's Color Director Louis Licari provides a full spectrum of do's and don'ts for tinting, highlighting, and shading your hair.

TALKING TO YOUR STYLIST

The first step toward making a positive change in your hair is to get the right cut. That doesn't mean throwing your hands up in the air and praying for a stylist who happens to do your hair beautifully that day. Every now and then you could get lucky, but don't bet your tresses on it. You must be able to tell the stylist what you want.

Magazine photos of a style you like can help, but too often what looks marvelous on the model comes out disastrous on you. The model's entire face and type of hair could be different. The same holds true for great cuts your friends might be sporting. Try to ask for something that fits what you have to work with.

One thing you have to discuss is the texture of your hair. Sure, everybody recognizes the difference between fine and coarse or curly and wavy. The trick here is to accept your hair for what it is. You have to be aware of your hair's limitations.

We all know women with fine, straight hair that insist on getting tight, tortured curls. I used to do the opposite. Years ago, I was one of those crazies who regularly ironed out the waves. Either way, it's self-defeating to ask a stylist to do things with your hair that go against its natural tendencies. Some pros will save you with a staunch refusal. But why risk it?

Pointing out facial flaws to your stylist is also worthwhile. However, it's wrong to demand a whole hairstyle that revolves around hiding a prominent nose. Ignoring the total look could throw everything out of balance. Most nose, forehead, or neck complaints can be minimized with some minor hair tricks that fit into an overall scheme.

Sometimes we communicate things to the stylist that interfere with what we really want. Don't try to make your present hairdo seem fabulous on the day you're going to the salon. You'll only be sending the stylist a subconscious message that begs for the same cut all over again. Walk in there with your hair flat and unstyled! Now she or he has to either listen carefully to your requests or use imagination to create something new.

Of course, your prime concern is to come up with a cut that's compatible with your face shape. Any hairstyle you select must be aimed at the ultimate oval. What's chic or up-to-the-minute doesn't mean a thing if it widens an already round face. In the next section we'll take a look at some styles that are ideal for the different face shapes. By the time we're through, you'll not only be recommending an appropriate cut to your stylist, you'll be describing it in concise professional terms.

Hairstyles for your face shape

Let's do a lightning-fast appraisal of your present hairstyle. Step in front of your makeup mirror with your hair pulled back. This will allow you to reaffirm once again the geometry of your face. Now, comb your hair in the usual manner. Repress the urge to self-consciously puff it up or slick it down.

Does your face suddenly seem ovalized, thinner, or better proportioned? If the reply is no, then brace yourself for some radical changes. You're going to be *contouring* the shape of your face by rearranging your hair. That's right—many of the contouring tricks used in the makeup chapter can be adapted to the way you cut and comb.

Remember how a darker foundation caused certain areas of your face to be overlooked or recede? Well, hair of almost any color gives a similar effect by covering up a part of your forehead or jawline. Push your hair away from the borders of your face, and you highlight an area just as a lighter foundation did. The biggest difference is that hair can also be gathered above and to the sides of your face, which allows you to change the shape even more.

Contouring with medium-length or shorter hair is especially effective. From the chin upward you soften the lines of the face as you rework the shape. The results are more pronounced because light shines through, separating your shoulders from where your hair-framed face begins. Study the following suggestions and decide which one does the most for the shape of your face.

The round face

Usually a round face sits atop a rather circular body. Therefore, you should avoid slimming your face so much that it makes the body seem even rounder by comparison. Our object here is to slightly narrow your face and at the same time make it appear a bit longer.

Your first move is to create some "accents" around the sides of your face. *Accent pieces* are strands of hair cut or feathered over areas

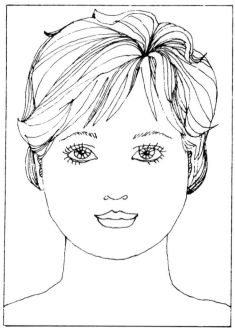

ROUND FACE, SHORT HAIR

that are too wide. These generally help to ovalize the face when the forehead is left clear. Some volume on the sides with a gradual mushrooming as you approach the crown adds to the effect. But don't end up with bubble styles that only increase the sense of roundness.

I find the *bob* to be a particularly good style for a round face. Women with sort of wavy medium-length or shortish hair should consider it strongly. It uses a full, even line of hair that stops at about center cheek. The idea is to boldly cut into the face and break up the width. You'll love how easy it is to comb and keep up. Plus, it's one of those beautiful classics that always manages to stay in vogue.

Another standard solution to the overly round shape is a *layered cut* that sweeps away from your face. Layering refers to cutting the top hairs shorter and making the hair progressively longer as you go down. These layers give you a soft fullness throughout. We also include a few accents to contour the cheeks. More volume in the back of the head balances out the style.

Stylist Kim Lepine believes most types of short hair need a layered look with soft side fringes to fit the round face. She feels long hair can benefit a round shape only when it's cut "blunt" and layered. A *blunt cut* means you shear off all the ends evenly with a scissor—no tapering of individual strands. Each hair must be as thick at the end as it is at the base.

The square face

Your square face boasts hard corners at the forehead and along the jaw. We want to ovalize your face by filling in those corners

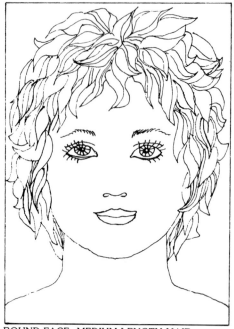

ROUND FACE, MEDIUM-LENGTH HAIR

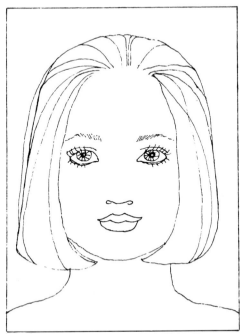

SQUARE FACE, MEDIUM-LENGTH HAIR

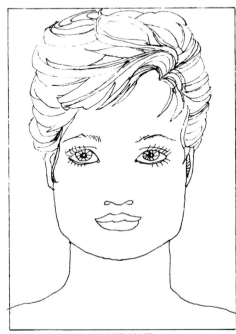

SQUARE FACE, SHORT HAIR

with a soft covering of hair. With long or medium-length hair you can hide all four corners. But short hair can still work by drawing attention away from the lower part of your face.

A great way of handling short hair on a square face is to put some eye-catching fullness on top. At the same time, we keep the sides close and the back fairly short. Fringy pieces on the perimeter of your face, starting at mid-cheek, further mold and soften those harsh angular lines. Wavy and curly hair will look better if the whole thing is layered. Fine hair requires less wispy, cleaner lines.

I think a *pageboy* is a good hairdo for medium-length hair. The pageboy is considered a "blunt style," which is more than just a blunt cut. This means all hair appears to be the same length and stops at the same place. At the bottom everything is still cut in a straight line. It's the thick, uniform ends of the pageboy that conceal the corners of your jaw and oval out the lower portion of your face. In addition, a hint of bangs get visibly longer as they move out to the sides. These spill over your temples. In the back, your hair should reach to about the middle of your neck.

If the pageboy seems too severe for you, go for a fluffier style. Comb a layered cut away from your face in broad, expansive strokes. It works just as well on the square face as it does on the round. However, the square face can take much more fullness on the sides. Be daring with this one! You could further soften those sharp cheekbones with a few feathered accents.

Women with long hair and a square face have very little room for fancy maneuvers.

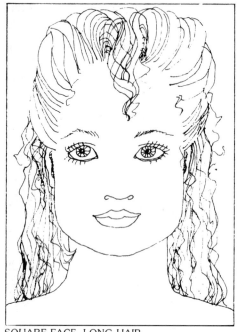

SQUARE FACE, LONG HAIR

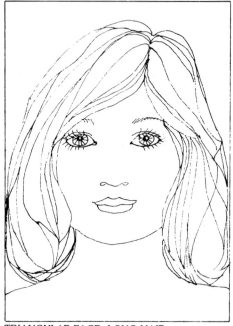

TRIANGULAR FACE, LONG HAIR

Kim sees the blunt style as their one safe alternative. Yet, a wavy or curly texture might get away with a layered cut. Long hair can also be a plus for those of you who want to wear it up. Hair worn above the square face requires a lot of volume on top and in the back of the head.

The triangular face

An extremely narrow forehead is the biggest problem for a triangular face. It has to be built up so it appears to balance out heavy cheeks and a wide chin area. Women with a medium length can create this fullness by *sweeping* hair from one side of the forehead to the other. The horizontal flow and volume form a startling illusion. Short fringes on the sides help to thin the cheeks just a smidgeon.

Short or medium-length hair that's too fine for the sweep might require a *permanent* for extra body. I'll show you how to do it later on in this chapter. Those of you with straight hair should also consider a shortish pageboy with bangs. Just don't make the hair on the bottom super thick.

Long hair that's straight or coarse can be done in a blunt style with accents along the sides. Wavy or curly hair looks better on a triangular face when it's layered. Here soft, wispy fringes go a long way. Don't try any kind of an upsweep with this face shape. We need all the hair we can muster to fill out the forehead and carve into those plump cheeks.

The diamond face

Cover up the wide, sharply pointed cheeks and soften the narrow, pointy forehead. That's all it takes to ovalize the diamond-shaped face. Actually, it's simple enough for women with short or medium-length hair. But forget about pulling out a winning oval with long hair. Any hair below your cheeks just accentuates the pointy chin and blows the whole thing.

Medium and shorter lengths do well with a loosely tousled, layered style. There should be a definite fullness at the temples and on the top. Accents over the cheeks provide a gentler slope to the sides of your face. Short, wispy bangs subtlely mute the center of your forehead. All attention is now directed away from the pointy chin. Again, women with fine strands can change the texture of their hair with a permanent.

The heart-shaped face

My face, for better or worse, is treated like a heart shape when it comes to hairstyles. The main objective is to cover my temples and generally reduce the size of my broad forehead. Like the diamond-shaped face, the heart's chin is quite pointy. So, I need a style that tends to equalize the top and bottom of my face. Not always an easy task!

My shortish, wash-and-wear cut is layered into a sea of natural waves. The fringe across my forehead falls over my temples and gets tucked behind my ears. I like to let my classy cheekbones show. Accents around my ears narrow things a bit more. And I don't bother to break up the effect with a part. It just looks that much more outdoorsy this way.

Right now, I'm seriously considering growing out my hair to a medium length. I'll keep it short on top and let the back get somewhat longer. It will still be layered, but I can try more

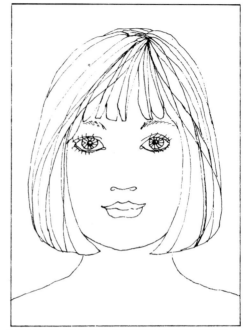

TRIANGULAR FACE, MEDIUM-LENGTH HAIR

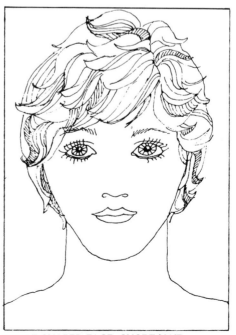

HEART-SHAPED FACE, SHORT HAIR

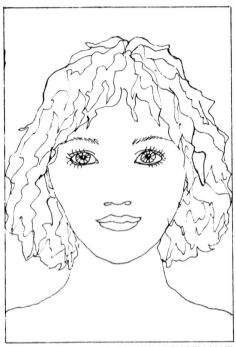

HEART-SHAPED FACE, MEDIUM-LENGTH HAIR

dramatic styles from time to time. I know it sounds silly to fidget with a good thing, but change can also be a good thing!

Women with a fine, coarse, or straight texture might prefer the bob for their middle-length hair. It should work well so long as there are a few accent pieces in the temple area. Try to make these accents asymmetrical so that the total appearance doesn't seem so pat. On the whole, hair should not extend all the way to your chin.

The *shag* look is another possibility for the heart-shaped face. For best results, maintain a fullness midway down and near the bottom. Hair covering the temples is essential. When done correctly, it's a hip, sensual style.

The heart-shaped face does not handle up-above-the-head styles or long, straight cuts very well. Both of these do nothing to solve imbalances. In fact, they only magnify the shortcomings. Long wavy and curly hair can be passable in a graduated cut. A blunt style will help long fine, medium coarse, or even straight hair. But the sides must be pulled away from your heart-shaped face to work.

STYLING TO FIX
OR ENHANCE YOUR FEATURES

Certain facial features that detract from your overall beauty can be remedied with very minor hair adjustments. These hair tricks should combine with makeup touches to create more convincing illusions. The key here is in not going overboard. These should all fit into your favorite style, which was determined by your face shape and hair texture.

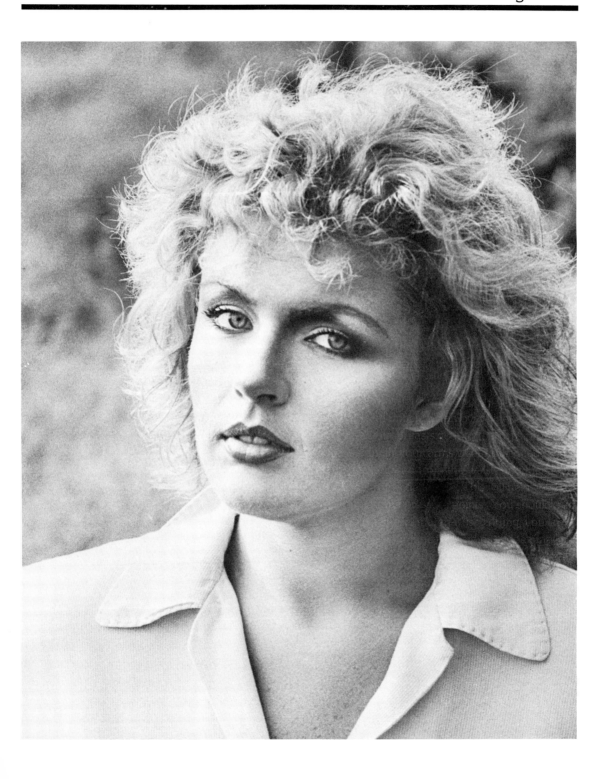

In fact, sometimes it's what you don't do that makes the biggest difference.

Prominent noses can be helped with some volume on top and in the back of the head. Almost any length will work. But don't go for a flat top or heavy fringes. Please, nothing too geometric either.

High foreheads must be covered to some degree by a fringe or bangs. Never wear your hair back off your face. And absolutely avoid that tight, pulled-back look.

Small foreheads can take soft, very wispy fringes. When possible avoid fringes altogether. Of course, don't even think about having heavy bangs.

Double chins look ten times worse when you wear a long pageboy. This style curves in under the jawline and terribly emphasizes the chin. Always make sure your hair ends before reaching the chin area. Better yet, try not to have any hair between your jawline and shoulders.

Extra-long necks must get some hair down the back and sides to look good. You'll need enough length to cover most of the neck. Don't attempt any close-cropped pixie cuts.

Short necks should have hair tapered in the back. Covering the neck totally or wearing your hair up on top of your head is also acceptable. However, a geometrically cut back is forbidden for less than swanlike necks.

Along with the features that need fixing there are a few attributes that require highlighting. Here are some ways to play up your assets.

Pretty eyes should be framed with accents. Try to draw attention to the center of the face. Avoid long bangs or sweeps that hide any part of your eyes or brows.

Prominent cheekbones best not be covered up. Take your hair away from the sides of your face. Accents above the cheeks can be effective if done gingerly and well.

Clean or straight hairlines are often hidden from view by women who don't appreciate what they have. Just ask a friend with an exaggerated widow's peak how important a straight hairline can be. For heaven's sake, show it off! Wear your hair up or away from your face. Avoid bangs, fringes, and wispy accents if possible.

WHEN TO CUT YOUR HAIR

Asking your stylist for that first image-changing cut is a big step. But once that's done you should have some practical game plan for keeping your hair in shape and at the best possible length. Knowing how your hair grows and when to get it cut is essential. The following are a few basic facts supplied by Kim Lepine.

☐ Hair grows about 1/2 inch to 1 inch a month.

☐ Hair sometimes goes through shock two to four days after a haircut. A day or so later your hair will become manageable again.

☐ Your hair should be cut every four to twelve weeks.

Four to five weeks All hair that's very fine, weak or colored with a chemical process. Hair that takes a permanent, relaxer, or is externally dry should also be cut in this time period.

Five to eight weeks Cut hair that's hard to

manage at this interval. This is also a good time frame for hair that has to be kept strictly in a certain style.

Eight to twelve weeks When letting your hair grow or if your hair is long and healthy take all the time you need. You'll look great even after that rough ten-week mark.

BODY BUILDERS FOR
YOUR HAIR

There are times when our physiques look tired, weak, or just plain flat. The solution is usually some kind of body-building or energizing program. Well, your hair might also appear lifeless and rundown every now and then. Chemical waves and sets will make your hair appear healthier. But they can sometimes do more harm than good. So, I recommend that you try some nonchemical body builders when your hair has the blahs.

The five-minute body set

For this instant remedy you'll need two special items. First get a plastic headband that's wide enought to reach from ear to ear. Then select any setting lotion from the many on the market. All of them are relatively gentle and quite safe.

Now spray the top and sides of your hair with water. Follow up by respraying your hair with some setting lotion. Gently comb your hair straight back, then slip the headband into place, and wait approximately five minutes until your hair dries. When you lightly brush your hair it will look soft, springy, and very alive.

Curlier hair without stress

Your hair might look something like mine—waves or loose curls coming out naturally. There's nothing wrong with that! But, we all occasionally envision a head full of tightly bunched curls. You can simply get the results you want by using those familiar pink sponge rollers that can be bought in almost any five-and-dime or drugstore. The real secret is knowing exactly how to use them.

If you check the displays, you'll see that there are four different sizes. Choose the one that's best for your hair length and desired tightness of curl. A light spray of setting lotion before using the rollers promises you a tighter curl. That same spray can also give curling power to straight or fine hair.

To set the top and sides of your head, hold the rollers close to your scalp. This is not the usual technique, but it's suitable for our specific aims. Wind your hair slowly around the sponges without yanking. And then fasten the rollers over the curls.

Setting the back of your hair begins with a more conventional approach. You roll all the hair from the ends toward the roots. The trick here is to twist the long strands prior to doing the roll. I also make a point of stopping the rollers about an inch or two before the roots. This prevents the fasteners from leaving nasty ridges.

Some women have curly hair that's too short for using sponge rollers. Don't feel cheated if you're one of them. Your curls can still get enough body to stand away from your head in a stylish bounce. Just wash your hair and moisten your fingertips with setting lotion.

Then quickly run your fingers through your damp hair; lift those natural curls and scrunch them with your lotioned fingers until everything dries. It makes a great evening look!

Black women with a fine, coarse, or medium texture might want to go in the other direction with their frizzy hair. Relaxers actually reduce the width of your roots. By relaxing certain areas you can create small, manageable curls. There are some very good hair relaxers on the market, but since this can be a fairly dangerous chemical process, I think going to an expert is the wisest thing to do.

Handling home permanents

In the past, home permanents have been shot-in-the-dark, risky treatments. Many women tried to stagger through them without knowing what to do and not really sure what to expect. Well, you're still better off going to a salon, but some high-quality, gentle home perms are now available. So, if you insist on making heavy-duty waves at home, at least let me give you a quick hair-saving orientation.

For openers, let's clear up some misconceptions about perms. It's not how long you leave the solution on your hair that determines the strength or size of the curl. The initial solution just changes the hair into a soft, shapeless substance. The perming really takes place when you rinse off the solution and apply the neutralizer. A neutralizer hardens the hair into whatever shape it's in at the moment. Hair wrapped around cylindrical rods obviously becomes circles.

When you remove the rods your hair forms a long chain of one S after another. These spirals are the permanent waves. The size of your waves is in proportion to the diameter of the rods you use. Very curly hair, therefore, requires the smallest possible rods. Large curls take medium-sized rods and an easy-flowing wave would call for giant rods.

Before dipping into the solution and rolling, consider the following suggestions.

☐ Don't do a home permanent by yourself. Have a wide-awake friend around to help you.

☐ Be sure to buy your own permanent rods. They'll give you a softer, more professional look than the ones supplied by the home-perm packages. And this way you get to choose the size of the rods.

☐ Plan in advance where you're going to put the rollers. Don't get impatient or you'll permanent wave areas that don't need it.

☐ Follow the directions on the package to the letter.

☐ Remember to use uniform sections around each rod so that you create a regular wave pattern.

☐ Make absolutely certain that the ends of your hair are neatly placed in the papers and wound around the rods. Not too tightly! This is where breakage, dryness, and fuzzy ends occur.

☐ Never do a permanent and coloring at home on the same day. You'll never get them right. In an emergency, go to a top salon. A talented stylist will get you through.

☐ One last *rule of thumb* should be said twenty times before every home permanent. Don't overdo it! You can always add more curls. But you can't undo a perm—short of cutting it all off. Aim for less.

Hair health tips

Sharp styling and substantial body give you aesthetically pleasing hair. But styles have to be kept up, and body needs new strength infused periodically. So above all, you have to keep your hair continually healthy.

My health tips fall into three fundamental categories: general hair care, when to condition your hair, and the use of hair appliances. These are sensible recommendations that give you a daily awareness of your hair's needs. You'll see that they often do more for your hair than the glamorous techniques.

General hair care

Here are a few facts, warnings, and hints to think about while you play with your beautiful new hairstyle.

□ Try to be as calm as you can. Nervous stress can hurt the health of your hair.

□ Check out thoroughly any medications you intend to use on your hair or scalp. Some medicines can severely damage follicles or roots.

□ Don't be afraid to shampoo as often as it takes to keep your hair clean. Experiment with mild shampoos that contain conditioners or dilute the stronger shampoos made strictly for cleaning.

□ Use hair accessories to support and structure long manes. Again, not too tight! Also avoid straining roots with naked rubber bands—get the covered variety.

□ Stick to a wide-toothed comb for untangling gnarled hair. It's the best way to escape breaking or pulling out your hair.

□ Eat a well-balanced diet! Even hair has to be properly nourished.

When to hair condition

Conditioning your hair has become as routine as washing your face. It's the easiest way to get extra body or manageable hair on a regular basis. Most conditioners are safely non-alkaline and pH balanced. But too much hair conditioning with the wrong kind of product can do you more harm than good. Follow a conditioning schedule that fits your hair texture.

Normal or medium-textured hair should be conditioned every other shampoo. An instant conditioner that can be rinsed out right away is sufficient. This will allow you to just zip a comb through your hair when you're finished.

Dry, coarse, and frizzy hair gets a conditioning with every single shampoo. Try the thicker, creamier conditioners, which have more power. If your hair feels greasy or appears stringy at the end of the day, your conditioner is just a little too heavy and is attracting dirt from the air. Switching to a slightly lighter conditioner will clear up the problem.

Fine hair that's on the dry side also has to be conditioned each time you shampoo. But the steps are a bit more complex. Begin by shampooing and rinsing your hair normally. Then put on a light conditioner for the time specified on the label. Certain noninstant products usually require five to ten minutes for maximum results. When you're ready, rinse out the conditioner and apply another small amount of shampoo. One last extensive rinse completes the process.

Oily hair has the distinction of never needing a conditioner. In fact, you'll only make the problem worse by using one.

Combination hair has oily roots and dry ends and demands some partial conditioning. Treat only the ends of your hair with a milder brand. Limit the conditioning to every second shampoo.

Using hair appliances

Electricity and hair don't really mix. Even friction sparks can make your hair stand on end. Yet you can do some marvelous things quickly with hot brushes or blowers. Just be sure you learn how to work these appliances and what to watch out for. And please don't do anything to excess!

Blow dryers These must be heat controlled like any other hair appliance. You should have at least three settings—hot, medium, and low. Always keep the dryer about six inches from your hair. Dryers can singe your hair and cause split ends when they're used at too close a range.

Begin drying a very wet head with hot air. Turn down to medium heat in a few moments and then soothe your damp hair with a low-temperature breeze. Long or thick hair dries faster if you bend over while using the blower. Finally, resolve to flick off the dryer before your hair is bone dry.

Electric rollers and curling irons Please, don't use these hot items every time you plan to step out of the house. When the juice *is* on, try not to put too much tension on your roots. Also, watch the clock to avoid overdoing, and remove the rollers very gently. You might even consider investing some time and money in an especially manageable hairstyle. This way you can forget about buying these appliances in the first place.

Hot brushes Quite a few styles get a lift from the heated bristles of a hot brush, which allows you to pull off a lot of fancy little styling tricks. However, go easy on yourself. Use a brush with widely-spaced bristles and keep it on the lowest setting that's effective for your hair. Don't be tempted to use the hot brush on a daily basis.

EXPERT COLOR CHANGES

Years ago, women had a rough time deciding whether or not to touch up their hair. Most took the coloring plunge only when the clock forced them to "get the gray out." Today, changing the shade of your hair is hardly the question. Women switch colors to make their hair seem livelier, a bit warmer, or just different than the month before.

Smart fuller-figure women can even use hair coloring like makeup. A few lighter tones around your forehead opens up that area, making your face appear to be slightly longer. For a narrower-looking face, simply darken the sides and lighten the hair on the top of your head. You can even draw attention away from double chins and close-set eyes.

Finding reasons to color hair is certainly easy enough. Today women seem more concerned about whether to do the transformation at home or in a salon. I happen to think there's a lot to be said in favor of professional direction. I've been known to drastically alter the color of my hair at home. Sometimes the results are a knockout. But too often I wind up, as many others do, in the colorist's chair asking for emergency repairs.

A good colorist is aware of what's right for your hair and your face. He or she will try to work with your natural hair color. Pros know which colors can be safely introduced without dulling the hair and what techniques produce the effect you need. It's that first decision-making session where the colorist is as valuable as a stylist. Later on, you should be able to do most of your own coloring fix-ups alone.

Questions to ask your colorist

Going to a top colorist is comparable to visiting a good medical specialist. Time is short and the bill is big. So, be prepared to ask the questions that really matter. Consider the condition of your hair, what might be done to it, and what you can expect afterward. Take into consideration your lifestyle and personal preferences when it's time for choosing. Try these questions on for starters and add anything *you* think is important:

□ What hair colors are compatible with my natural color? Jot down the choices. Ask for descriptions of colors that sound unfamiliar.

□ What is the present condition and quality of my hair? Will further chemical treatments be harmful? Ask which techniques are both gentle enough and still effective.

□ Will the color wear too fast? This refers to how quickly your new color will oxidize.

Will it wear gracefully? Now you're checking to see if the new color will oxidize to an acceptable shade.

□ How much of a commitment is necessary to maintain my new hue? Different colors or techniques take varying amounts of upkeep. Check to see if you have the time, money, or desire to make the change worthwhile.

□ What method of coloring suits my needs best?

Only after asking all the questions can you settle on a procedure. Modern hair coloring is an exact science that takes in everything from tinting to frosting. Each looks different, and some have stiffer consequences for mistakes.

Home hair coloring kits

A good colorist is a fine crutch, but these specialists are rare outside the largest cities. Usually your stylist will double as a color consultant. To be on the safe side you should be able to change and retouch your hair color at home. With this in mind, La Coupe's Louis Licari has helped me put together coloring survival hints for home use. We want you to get a sense of what is fact and what is fiction.

Most home coloring kits are extremely potent. This is to guarantee that they work. Most customer complaints are caused by processing. So be careful about which color you pick and how much you use. Stay close to your natural color to avoid colors that turn later.

Once you've chosen a shade it's best not to leave the solution on the full thirty minutes. "What you'll get is a more translucent rather than opaque hair color," says Louis. "You'll be letting some of your real color show through, which means the natural nuances and shine of your hair is preserved." In other words, it'll look like your true color and not something poured out of a bottle.

Home highlighters

Home use of highlighters should also be underdone. They are strong chemical lighteners designed to brighten up a few selected strands here and there. Medium-brown to blond hair is supposed to get a sun-bleached quality from home highlighters. Unfortunately, any mistakes made with these peroxide products can't be washed away. Go too far and you'll need scissors or lots of growing-out time to get back to where you started.

The secret is in knowing the potential of your original color. Chemical highlighting can have some strange effects on certain shades. For instance, dark-brown hair is often streaked orange by highlighters. I don't recommend doing it at home. Ash-blond or some kinds of light-brown hair can develop a greenish tint in the wrong light. And highlighters left too long on blond hair give you an absolutely lifeless white-blond.

Yet, many women with brown or blond hair wind up with some beautiful results from highlighting. Try to gradually let the small sections of your hair lighten to a golden stage. Gold isn't the brassy look that we've been programmed to run away from. Yellow, red, and gold are the highlights found in a child's hair. These are the highlighting colors that we want because they can reflect light and give off a shine. All other artificial shades absorb the light and appear lackluster.

LOUIS'S NATURALLY SAFE
HOME HIGHLIGHTERS

We seem to have a highlighting dilemma shaping up here. Going to a salon for highlighting is safe but for some, means too much of a fuss and expense. Home highlighting products are cheaper, more convenient, but, alas, riskier. What's a confused Big Beauty to do?

Louis Licari has an answer that offers the best of both worlds. He suggests a leisurely shampoo at home followed by a *highlighter rinse*. These are natural, water-based colors mixed up in your own kitchen. They work slowly to bring out richer highlights and shine in any color hair. And mistakes here can be solved with some more shampooing.

Pick out the natural highlighter from these three recipes that cater to your hair color. The results you can expect are listed after each one. Oh, yes, women with chemically treated hair should wait two weeks after their treatment before using rinses.

RECIPE 1

8 tablespoons of chamomile
1 quart of water
Boil water and let chamomile simmer in a covered pot for twenty minutes. Strain and cool before using.

RESULTS: If you have *medium to dark-brown hair* you'll develop auburn highlights with consistent applications.

Light-brown to dark-blond hair will become blonder and, natural highlights will be brought out after several rinses.

Any *brown hair with natural or processed highlights* will have those areas brightened.

RECIPE 2

10 tablespoons of hibiscus
1 quart of water
Boil water and let covered ingredients simmer one full hour. Strain and cool liquid.

RESULTS: Your *auburn hair* will get slightly redder.

Brown hair with blond highlights will have those highlights turn gradually to a strawberry blond.

Light to dark blonds can develop strawberry-blond highlights.

RECIPE 3

Shells from 1 pound of walnuts
1 quart of water
First broil the shells until they're brown. Grind brown shells in food processor. Now boil water and simmer shells in covered pot for two hours. Strain and cool the liquid.

RESULTS: Expect *black or brunette hair* to turn darker and richer.

Brown with gray hair mixed in can have gray areas darkened to look more like highlights.

HENNA AND OTHER LEMONS

I just want to add a quick word about other fabled, natural highlighters. All through the seventies and into the eighties, henna was touted as a miracle dye harvested from the leaves of a wild shrub. It was supposed to safely give your hair extra shine, brightness, conditioning, holding power, and lightness. Don't believe the myth just because it screams N-A-T-U-R-A-L!

The truth is henna doesn't match up well to many of the manufactured hair colors around today. Henna is as strong as any chemical coloring on the market, but isn't as gentle as quite a few. If you put henna over already colored hair it would only make everything duller. What's more, henna makes permed hair heavier and loosens the wave. And, just for the record, henna isn't a lightener or a conditioner.

A no-peroxide hair color rinse is probably safer and more accurate in achieving what you thought henna could do. Yet, some people can benefit from henna. It's good for women with fine, oily hair, since it is very heavy in protein and acts as a powerful sealer.

Okay, I promised you other lemons. Well, they're yellow and make your mouth pucker and really do give your hair highlights. In tales of ancient beauties, there's even talk about how Venetian women pulled strands through straw hats and squeezed lemon juice on them. Then they'd go out into the sun until the exposed hairs lightened. Lemons were sort of a natural frost-and-tip kit in biblical times.

You'll be much better off believing and learning from my little lemon story than getting stuck with a lemon like henna!

CHAPTER SEVEN

FULLER-FIGURE FASHION: A BRAVE NEW WORLD

Up until a few years ago I did most of my clothes shopping in men's stores. I know that's not *so* unusual. Even the skinniest girls like to throw on a man's shirt once in a while. But for me this was fashion survival rather than a dress-up whim. At the women's shops, I could never find decent styles in my size made of nonpolyester fabrics.

Oh, it was murder standing elbow to elbow on Saturday mornings with guys rummaging for the right slacks or jeans. There's something disturbing about holding a pair of jeans up to your waist that the burly man next to you just put down. However, the biggest embarrassment usually came after finding the pants I was looking for. Men's clothes are cut narrow to hug those slim-hipped creatures. So, if I got

jeans that fit my broad hips the waist would be gigantic. And the cashier always did a long double take while folding them into the bag.

Those were the days when the Lords of Fashion only smiled on women wearing a small dress size. Larger gals had nothing new, little choice, and loads of tailoring to do on whatever they decided to buy. In addition, most bright colors, fairly interesting patterns, and sexy styles never made it to the fuller-figure racks. If my mother hadn't taught me to sew I probably would've drowned in baggy material and the nothing-to-wear blues.

Today, there's a brave new fashion world for the size 16 and over. Manufacturers are just starting to realize that large women equal big business and enormous profits. Major department stores now publicize growing sections dedicated to our needs. Sure there's still a sprinkling of polyester in their inventory. But for the most part these superstores are going with younger styles, more flattering fabrics, and colorful designs.

Yet you must be strong, even insistent, about requesting styles and clothing lines you admire. Many of these departments are fighting budget problems. Your demands will let management know that more funds are needed to properly stock large-sized areas. Also, the clothes you ask for will make it clear that tunics and tent dresses are not enough. *You* have to help create the new awareness!

By the way, there are a lot of fuller-figure boutiques popping up around the country. These places concentrate only on our size range and are tuned into the latest breakthroughs. They also tend to employ other large ladies as salespeople. Unfortunately, small specialty shops almost always have to charge more than the huge department stores, but the quality and variety are worth a little more.

Getting access to stylish clothes is only half the fashion struggle. You also have to throw out all the forbidding myths, nagging doubts, and outdated notions about dressing a large body. Cultivate an open-minded approach and knowing eye instead, and take a few smartly planned chances!

I'm aware that neither confidence nor knowledge comes without some effort. So, I'm going to make things somewhat easier by explaining how to put together a complete wardrobe. I'll show you the art of rack picking along with the basics of home sewing.

You'll get a feel for what fits your size and beautifies your specific body type. In no time you'll be glamorously dressed from fine undergarments to a *trés chic* overcoat.

OUT-OF-SIGHT FASHION

The blueprint for assembling any fuller-figure outfit has to begin with a good *foundation*. I'm referring to all the unmentionables that are supposed to hold you up, keep you in, or smooth you out. Sure, they're hidden beneath a layer of fabric in public. But the wrong ones can stand out more than an ostrich-plumed hat. These are the monstrous contraptions that openly distort your body and leave a pained expression on your face.

Large women have been torturing themselves with viselike bras, girdles, and corsets for generations. One of these martyrs was singer-actress Lillian Russell. Back in the Gay Nineties she earned the title of The American Beauty by rearranging her bountiful figure with a *wasp-waist* corset. When Lillian dined with Diamond Jim Brady, her midsection was so tightly cinched that her breasts bulged upward while her hips were forced down and out. The effect was grossly unnatural. And more than one evening was spent trying to ignore cracked ribs.

Today, there are still women who insist on wearing heavy, harmful foundations. Thick-ribbed corsets with broad lacing and triple panels of Lycra are all too common. I've also seen whole stores filled with big-boned longline bras and life-squeezing panty girdles. Some of these panty girdles can create enough pressure to badly damage internal organs. If you haven't got a back problem or some other congenital weakness, then it's time to stop strapping yourself into such severe forms of support.

I want you to seek out bras and body firmers that go lighter on your physique. After all, we're living in an era that calls for active, energetic women. You should be asking for undergarments that fit correctly, look natural, and allow you to move freely. Avoid putting yourself in a position where each motion pinches, pulls, or tightly binds.

A bra for all reasons

When shopping for a brassiere keep your complete life-style in mind. A clear evaluation might prompt you to buy more than just one type of bra, just as you wouldn't expect one dress to accommodate every occasion. Nobody wears last night's leather heels to jog around the block. So why limit yourself to the same old bra no matter what you're doing?

Try to match the features of different bras to your specific activities. Take an *underwire bra* for example. With a regular cup this bra gives buxom women extra containment and separation for *everyday* use. Underwire bras also come with *minimizer cups* to make you appear smaller on top. I personally don't approve of minimizers because they harshly flatten you down while pushing the extra flesh out to the sides. It just doesn't look right.

On the sporting scene you should switch to a bra that moves with your body. A *running bra* can't have underwires or even seams. The stitching along a seam could irritate your nipple. However, the straps are wider and more

rigid to prevent constant bouncing. Good *tennis bras* also have broader straps that meet in a V-back design. These straps won't slip off your shoulders in the middle of a volley, and the flexible material stretches every time you bend for a short ball or reach for a high one.

Certain bras are even made to complement particular outfits in your closet. For instance, the *plunge bra* is perfect for anything with a scandalously low neckline. It's cut to show you off without being seen. Yet, some of these front-hooking bras can be painfully binding around the midriff on large women. Look for the ones that are well designed.

Bras with a *seamless, molded cup* do quite a bit for knit dresses, sweaters, or sheer blouses. There are no telltale ridges to ruin the smooth effect, and the fabric conforms to your shape within a half hour after putting it on. Actually, fuller-figure gals should hold out for the ones with polyester fiberfill side panels. Those inserts help to support the weaker areas where your breasts lose elasticity first.

Women who must have maximum body control can add a *long-line brassiere* to the collection. Please, get the filleted variety that comes without big ominous bones. Also, to be really comfortable, a long-line must be geared to the length of your waist. Measure from under your bustline to your natural waistline. If the tape reads three inches or less, you're short-waisted and require a short model. A three- to five-inch count translates into a three-quarter-length bra; five to seven inches means you take a long, and over seven inches falls into the extra-long size range.

A recent manufacturing feat has finally produced a *strapless underwire bra*, made completely of Spandex, that is everything a fuller-figure woman has dreamed about. In general, check to see if a bra has a curved leotard back. This stops the fabric from digging into your flesh, because it flexes with the contour of your body. Soft cups should be reinforced with elastic underneath to cut down on curling. And underwire bras must have the wires recessed to effectively prevent them from popping.

FITTING YOUR BRA

Recognizing the kind of brassiere you want and the features you prefer won't mean much if the fit is off. Don't just hold up bras to your chest, rush through lightning try-ons, or read the labels. Instead, carefully follow this foolproof routine for finding an ideal fit.

1 Determine the *bra size* before going into the store. Essentially your bra size equals the circumference of the areas on a line with your upper back. You can get the exact circumference by running a tape measure under both arms and across the space above your breasts. Take any odd numbers and bring them up to the next even figure. For example, a 39-inch circumference means that you should purchase a size-40 bra. We always move toward more room to assure comfort.

2 Know the precise *cup size* you'll need to look and feel right. Here you have to measure the circumference of your chest by passing the tape directly over the fullest part of your bust. Now subtract your bra size from the bust measurement. Every inch left over equals a cup size. So, say your bra size is a 40 and your bust tallies 42 inches around. Those two surplus inches indicate that

you have a B cup. Three extra inches would tell you to get a C cup, four inches means a D cup, five inches a DD cup, and so on.

3 Try the brassiere on correctly and *check for balance*. Remember to lean over when you put on the bra so your breasts go into the cups properly. Once it's on lift your arms over your head, bend all the way forward from the waist, and then twist your body from side to side. This will help you find any troublesome pressure points. You should also note whether the material is binding you anywhere. Take your time in deciding. If the brassiere is right for you, the weight will be evenly distributed throughout the straps, cups, and overall construction.

Other body-saving foundations

A drawer full of great bras is only one step toward building a foundation that both controls and caresses your whole body. Now it's time to burn that iron-fisted corset, ban the treacherous panty girdle. Replace them instead with more modern kinds of apparel that allow you to slightly firm up your appearance without paying a painful price. Okay, ready to join the active eighties. Get yourself into one of these for a change:

BODY SUITS

These are sometimes called "all-in-ones." You're hugged gently by a continuous sheath of flexible material that goes from your shoulders down to the top of your legs. An added advantage is that a body suit has no unsightly breaks at the panties and bra. I recommend you wear the body suit under clothes that fit close to your skin, but don't try to jam it under outfits that are really tight. Box and barrel shapes can especially benefit from body suits with extra waist-firming strength.

PANTY BRIEFS WITH LYCRA

Don't let the word *Lycra* alarm you. When used wisely and in moderation Lycra can be both firm on your figure and soft on your skin. A light panty brief tends to smooth down the derriere, while mildly flattening your tummy. Barrel shapes with quite bulging stomachs should get a control brief that comes with an extra panel of Lycra. Believe me, that'll hold you in just fine.

PANTY GIRDLES

I used to wear one of these to hide my heavy thighs. All it did was give the appearance of sausage legs—ouch! Actually, I'm mentioning panty girdles here to remind you *not* to use them. Girdles hold you in so tightly that your muscles get lazy. In the long run your body has to control itself to some extent. Besides, girdles look terrible under slacks because the borders show through so blatantly.

BUSTIERS

Lillian Russell would have a grand old time in one of these playful things. A bustier is to-day's benevolent answer to her vicious wasp-waist corset. It's a strapless bra that continues down to gently cinch your waist and hold up your stockings. The bustier is usually worn with a low-cut evening dress or just to give the man in your life a lusty thrill. You don't wear it too often, but nobody forgets the bustier too quickly.

GARTER BELTS

Don't laugh! Here's an item that's coming back into style with a vengeance. They're fun and make it a lot easier to ditch that awful girdle. Be sure the top fits your waist, and remember to adjust the garters to the proper length. You don't want to feel them pressing into your fleshy thighs. And be a little daring with the styles you select.

Dazzling Daywear

Once you've laid the foundation it's smart to add a layer of silky things to act as a buffer. These are items that dress up the foundation and keep outer clothes from bunching or catch-ing. In the lingerie business such under-garments are called *daywear*. My daywear list for fuller-figure women includes slips, panties, camisoles, half slips, and teddies.

Up until a few years ago, daywear tended to turn all white, functional, and boring when it hit the larger sizes. Full slips, half slips, and camisoles came in plain white tricot. Take it or leave it! Teddies, featured in the begin-ning of Chapter 3, were clearly marked for skinnies only. We were deprived of the emo-tional lift that comes from draping a teddy under slacks or over often unsightly pantyhose.

Now, we have complete lines of daywear—exciting daywear—made ex-clusively for us. What a relief it is to choose from luscious ice-cream pastels or seductive designs in black. My lingerie is suddenly reflective of my moods, color coordinated, ex-tremely youthful, even amazingly varied.

SLIPS/CAMISOLES/TEDDIES

size	38	40	42	44	46	48	50	52
Fits bust	39-42	41-44	43-46	45-48	47-50	51-54	53-56	55-58
Fits waist	33-36	35-38	37-40	39-42	41-44	45-48	47-50	49-52
Fits hips	42-45	44-47	46-49	48-51	50-53	53-56	55-58	57-60
Dress size	16-18 or 38	18-20 or 40	20-22 or 44	22-24 or 44	46	48	50	52

HALF SLIPS

size	L	XL	XX	3X	4X
Fits waist	33-36	37-40	41-44	45-48	49-52
Fits hips	42-45	46-48	49-52	53-56	57-60
Dress size	18-20 or 38-40	20-22 or 40-42	22-24 or 42-44	46-48	50-52

PANTIES

size	9	10	11	12
Fits waist	33-36	37-40	41-44	45-48	49-51
Fits hips	43-46	46-49	49-52	52-55	55-58

What's more, all these goodies are durable and fit like an exotic dream. Skinnies, eat your hearts out!

Picking out colors and styles of lingerie is easy. You merely go for what pleases you. Finding the right size takes a bit more knowledge. I suggest studying these charts for a detailed analysis of what each size means.

PANTIES

Panties should get a special mention in this section. They are perhaps the most basic piece of clothing in your entire wardrobe.

Don't be embarrassed when you shop for them. Get some of the flamboyant patterns and shocking colors. Also, buy a style that makes sense for your body.

Briefs give you the most coverage. A quality brief will look fine under skirts, dresses, and some slacks. Those of you who are figure 8s or pears should make sure that the leg opening doesn't press against your flesh. This creates an obvious ridge where the panty hits the thigh.

Bikinis are okay if you get a really good, smooth fit. Don't wear any panty that allows flesh to overflow past the coverage points. Bikinis usually work best under a dress or skirt.

Once again, the right size is the key to success. Look over this chart before running to buy your new panties. By the way, those low numbers on panties are a great psychological lift.

FASHIONS FOR YOUR LEGS

Let's go from the totally out-of-sight fashions to a part of your wardrobe that alternates between invisibility and the center of attraction. I'm talking about the things you wear on your legs. Under a pair of pants your hosiery or socks are virtually hidden. But when you switch to a dress or skirt that legwear can often dominate a viewer's attention.

You don't quite believe me? Okay, go back and take a peek at the snapshot of yourself in street clothes. You remember, it was one of the photos from Chapter 3. You'll notice that approximately a third of your body is located below your waist. Good or bad, your legs are hard to overlook. It's up to you to decide whether they'll be working for or against you.

Fortunately, a substantial percentage of fuller-figure women are blessed with great gams. If you're one of the lucky ladies, I'll show you how to push those shapely legs into the spotlight as often as possible. Barrel types can especially benefit by playing up their thin legs. It's a fantastic way to take people's eyes off a rather thick middle. I'll also help those of you with stocky legs to put the focus elsewhere.

Hosiery — panty and otherwise

Nylon stockings have traditionally been the accepted approach to dressing up your legs. Since World War II, no woman over eighteen would dare to wear anything else with a skirt. But nowadays *pantyhose* have taken over at work or play. They combine the delicate beauty of nylons with the functional support of tights. All you have to do is decide which styles and color schemes are best for you.

For starters, pantyhose are fit to coincide with your height and weight. Every package of pantyhose has the appropriate chart on the back. This is in direct contrast with stockings, which are made to fit your shoe size and come in short, medium, long, and extra-long lengths. Whenever you're at the higher end of a pantyhose weight range, it's advisable to move up to the next size.

Each type of pantyhose seems to have certain pluses or minuses. You should look them all over and decide where your priorities lie. Here's the way I see them.

Sheer pantyhose These usually fit superbly. Sheer pantyhose stretch farther and easier than any other kind. Too bad their life expectancy is so short.

Ultrasheer pantyhose I won't bother with a durability rating. A bigger problem is the way they tend to bag at the ankles. And they just don't adjust easily to a large calf.

Support hose Most of these give you smooth, lively control. They seem to take a lot of pressure off your legs. Support hose last much longer than the sheer ones. I prefer to wear them under slacks for a rumple-free legline.

Tummy-control pantyhose It's a pleasant, but effective device for leveling off a bulging stomach. The negative aspect here is the cost. These pantyhose are expensive and can perish fairly quickly under the strain. A panty-control brief can do the same job for less money in the long run.

Hosiery hues for you

Once you've selected the style of pantyhose that fits your body and bankroll, it's time to concentrate on colors. Both pantyhose and regular hosiery are available in a multitude of shades and patterns. In fact, many of the hues found in pantyhose are offered in stockings. Your choice of colors should be dictated by whether you want to showcase your legs or leave them in the shadows.

HIGHLIGHTING PRETTY LEGS

Wear light-toned hosiery. Beige or nude stands out well without assaulting the eyes.

For dressier occasions you can come off quite chic by consciously blending the color of your stockings with the shade of your outfit. In general, mocha or off-gray go with most evening ensembles. Of course, when putting on the ritz you must go sheer.

Opaque hosiery can take center stage without really trying. Please, stick to the pale shades that will at least coexist with the rest of your attire. Once again, beiges and grays are safe. Bright colors turn opaque pantyhose into neon lights. All anyone will see coming are your high-voltage legs.

Patterns will get your legs noticed too. But remember, we're committed to good taste. Don't get too bold or flashy with the lines on your legs. Mesmerize the leg watchers by slipping into sheer hosiery adorned with fine designs, such as point d'esprit.

MUTING SHORT OR HEAVY LEGS

Fuller-figure women with a figure-8, pear-shape, or box-shape body very often have heavy thighs or calves. A few of these gals have short, stumpy legs, too. If you're in this category, take heart. You can minimize your leg flaws by toning down the hosiery you wear. Perhaps these suggestions will make a difference.

When wearing sheer hosiery stay away from pale shades. Medium tones are okay, but darker colors are much better. You'll find the really dark sheers slenderizing, maybe sexy as well.

Surprising as it seems, colorful opaque hosiery *isn't* out of the picture. But there's a definite catch: you must soften the opaque effect by keeping to the bleaker end of the colors available. I'd approve of navy, burgundy, brown, olive green, gray, and black.

Here's another shocker for you: certain patterns can also be worn successfully on chunky limbs. However, your choices are limited to fine pinstripes that come in low-profile monotones. Anything rowdier would badly hurt your fashion cause.

Socks and legwarmers

Our whole lives are not spent strutting around in nylons and pantyhose. Teens, sports enthusiasts of all types, and your everyday socks lovers would gladly tell you that. Both socks and legwarmers have become a regular part of the size-16-and-over getup. They're in vogue for large women because now we're more at ease and into physical games.

Barrel-shaped women probably get the biggest boost from knit legwear. You gals can scrunch legwarmers down over your calves and ankles when wearing jeans. This not only provides extra warmth in winter, but it helps to balance out the thinnest portion of your slender legs. Barrels can also put on just about any long socks with their skirts and loafers. Short socks teamed with running shorts or golf culottes look terrific too.

Pears, boxes, and figure 8s with shorter or huskier legs have to be a lot more selective. On tennis courts, bicycle paths, or jogging routes, only absorbent foot socks, or peds, will do. Anklets won't break up the line of your heavy calf well enough. Legwarmers for dancing or warm-ups are permissible, but don't let them bunch up. And any socks are fine for stuffing into boots.

Eye-catching dresses

Not too long ago, dresses were the accepted norm. Everything else was dubbed strictly casual, for specific occasions only, or just plain inappropriate. A woman's daily wardrobe was anchored by her front line of dresses. Sure, a couple of pairs of pants floated on the periphery; perhaps a suit or two got mixed in. But dresses were the mainstay.

In the eighties, dresses amount to just a few drops in closets that swim with diversity. So many worlds are open to us, and each creates another fashion twist. Yet, nothing makes you feel as wonderfully feminine as a flattering dress. It can buoy you up through an other-wise draggy day. A while later, with an accessory change, the same dress turns absolutely festive for the evening.

Our problem is finding those dresses that give us a personal lift. We've been out of touch with correct buying procedures for too long. Millions of large women don't completely understand the dress-sizing system or how to pick the styles that most improve their body shapes. Well, I'm ready to fill in the gaps for you.

About the size of it

Confusion about fuller-figure dress sizes stems from the three distinct categories being used: Misses, Half Sizes, and Women's Sizes. Each category is geared to service a large body with slightly different proportions than the other two. The criteria for the groupings remains fuzzy for many women. In addition, each category employs a separate numbering format, which drives most of us crazy. I remember times when size 18 would hang on me and a size-36 dress would be straining at the seams.

The best way to handle these categories is one at a time. I'll give the rationale for each, and you can decide which one is right for your body. It'll help if you're honest about your true height and body type. Some women might be able to find wearable items in more than one category.

MISSES OR WHOLE SIZES

This is the most recognizable and common category among the three. It's supposed to indicate dresses made for equally proportioned women of average height. That translates into

MISSES SIZES

size	16	18	20	22	24
Fits bust	37½–38½	39–40½	41–42½	43–44½	45–46½
Fits waist	29½–30½	31–32½	33–34½	35–36½	37–38½
Fits hips	40–41	41½–43	43½–45	45½–47	47½–49

HALF SIZES

sizes	14½	16½	18½	20½	22½	24½
Fits bust	37–38½	39–40½	41–42½	43–44½	45–46½	47–48½
Fits waist	31–32½	33–34½	35–36½	37–38½	39–41½	41½–43½
Fits hips	38–39½	40–41½	42–43½	44–45½	46–47½	48–49½

WOMEN'S SIZES

size	34	36	38	40	42	44	46
Fits bust	37–38½	39–40½	41–42½	43–44½	45–46½	47–48½	49–50½
Fits waist	31–32½	33–34½	35–36½	37–38½	39–41	41½–43½	44–46
Fits hips	38–39½	40–41½	42–43½	44–45½	46–47½	48–49½	50–51½

figure 8s and maybe a few box shapes standing from 5 feet 3½ inches to 5 feet 7 inches tall. You should therefore be neither top- nor bottom-heavy to fit comfortably into one of these dresses. The number range for fuller-figure sizes begins with 16 and goes up by twos: 16, 18, 20, 22, 24. See if your measurements match up with one of the sizes listed in the Misses chart.

HALF SIZES

Unlike Misses, this is a name that reveals an awful lot. First, it warns you that every number in the size listing has a half tagged on the end, such as 14½, 16½, 18½, 20½, and so on. The Half Sizes title tells you something about the dresses and the women in them. These dresses tend to have shorter waists, sleeves, and an overall length. Gals wearing Half Sizes are predictably under 5 feet 4 inches in their stocking feet. And, for some unknown reason, fashions in this category seem to be only half as youthful in design.

So, shortish pears and barrel shapes, brace yourselves. Prepare to make the best of a trying situation. Then, examine the Half Sizes chart to determine where your body fits in.

WOMEN'S SIZES

This third category is almost the opposite of the Half Sizes. Everything here is in terms of more rather than less. All Women's Sizes lean toward proportionately longer waists, sleeves, and total length. The women who use these

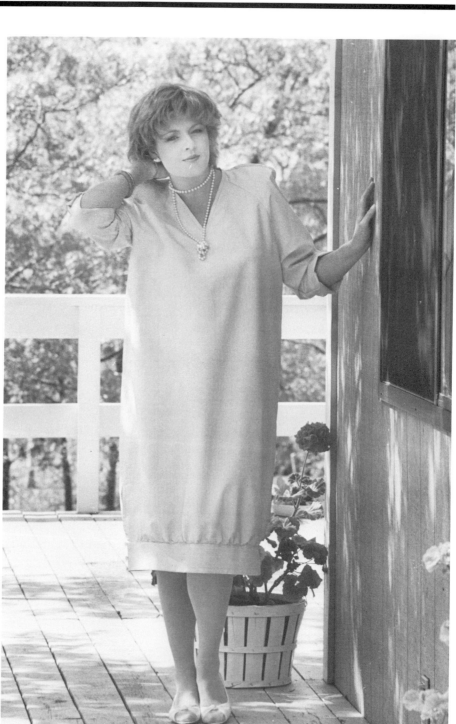

dresses are tall figure 8s or boxes towering over 5 feet 7½ inches. I fall into the Women's Sizes classification and find little to complain about. It's the most contemporary size range, with new creations being added regularly. In keeping with its image, the size range here starts at a higher number and goes up quickly by twos: 34,36,38,40,42, and right on into the 50s.

Don't let all this precision measuring throw you. The specifications on the size charts are generally representative of what's right for each category. However, some manufacturers do use slightly different sets of proportions. So be flexible if a dress you like has a size you didn't quite expect. It just might fit beautifully!

Your dress style

Charts steer you more or less to the correct size. But the route to an ideal style is sort of freewheeling. We're thankfully flooded with new, tantalizing fashions today. I see variations on old favorites, foreign influences, and seasonal offerings that come and go like time itself. You have to develop a sense of what's made for your body.

Obviously, I don't have the space to go over every single dress style with you. We'd need a separate book just for that. However, I can warn you about certain styles that are clearly no-nos for your body type. Better yet, I can give you a rundown of the kinds of dresses which fool an observer's eye. These dresses take attention away from your "problem zone" and create the illusion of body balance. Note which styles are recommended for your shape.

Chemise Here's a dress that's capable of hiding a multitude of sins. It's especially effective on boxes, barrels, and figure 8s. The chemise is a classic straight-up-and-down design, which gives you a uniformly thinner overall appearance. Barrels use it to hide the thickness around their middles. Box shapes merely add a belt to the chemise to form the impression of a waistline.

Yet smart women keep their chemise loose fitting and easy on the eyes. Try not to get one in a flashy color or big print. Look for lightweight fabrics that drape softly over your figure instead of clinging. I personally prefer to widen the shoulders of my chemise dresses with pads. It comes out a little more dramatic, and my hips seem to shrink by comparison.

Shirt dresses When you combine a shirt with a flair skirt it diverts all eyes away from overly full hips. This makes shirt dresses a natural for pears and boxes. You can further strengthen the diversion by having pretty details at work up above the waist. For instance, a tailored collar with a colorful bow does the trick. Those neck-high details also draw attention away from a pear's less-endowed chest.

Blouson styles Any billowy-topped dress is a godsend for both pears and boxes. The added puffs give a pear's torso just enough roundness to balance off the hips. That same puffiness brings an artificial waistline to the normally curveless box-shaped body. Once again, shoulder pads will tend to accentuate the effects you're after.

Dropped-waist dresses Figure 8s and boxes should use drop waists to break up their rigidly symmetrical lines. Imagine how sleek

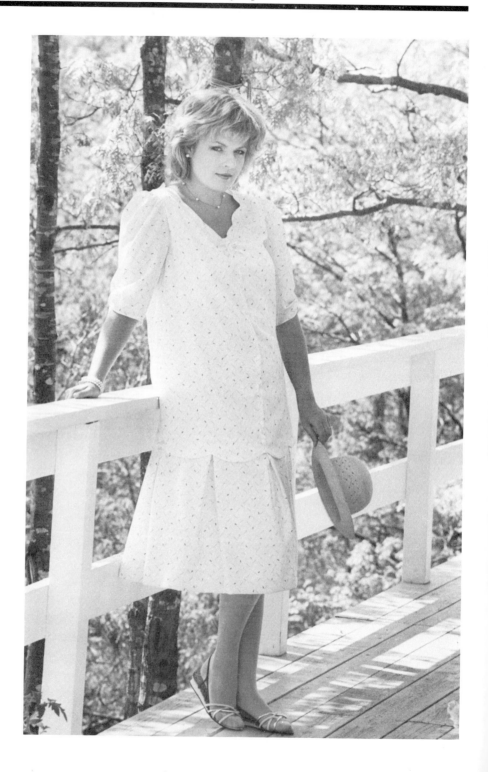

an hourglass-shape woman would look with seemingly pared down hips. Box shapes also lose some lower-torso bulk by creating a moderate indentation. These dresses are always comfortable and in very good taste.

Gala dresses I thought you might appreciate some pointers on what styles to wear for a superformal occasion. First of all, any kind of fuller-figure body is enhanced by a long nonbinding dress. Likewise, any large woman should avoid frilly things or heavy fabrics. Breezy simplicity is the essence of high fashion.

Figure 8s, pears, and boxes might want to substitute shoe-length skirts with alluring blouses. The lean legs of a barrel can even be covered by dressy pants. Before leaving be sure to study yourself from the back and sides in the mirror. After all, these are the parts of you everybody sees as you dance around the floor.

SUIT YOURSELF

Dresses make you feel like a woman, but they seem to be taking a back seat lately to more versatile suits. If a dress manages to trick the viewer's perception of your body one way, a suit enhances your proportions with several little illusions simultaneously. In traditional matching suits, made of an identical fabric throughout, you can play with the cut of the jacket as well as the skirt or pants. When you shop for a nontraditional suit, the possibilities really begin to multiply. Now you get to mix together tops and bottoms of different materials, patterns, colors, or textures.

Unfortunately, large women often don't end up taking advantage of what suits have to offer. Hardly any of us are able to recognize the combinations that glamorize our particular figures. Patterns, such as plaids, are either badly abused or rejected out of hand. Many smart styles are rather dumbly written off as being "for skinnies only." Why, some hefty gals I know still act positively horrified by the idea of wearing a velvet jacket over a wool skirt.

Stop depriving yourself of a potent fashion weapon. The elements for putting together a flattering suit are simple to apply. Light colors come forward and darker ones recede, just like they do in makeup. Busy patterns or textures draw attention, while flat solids tend to be overlooked. And jacket lengths or details can either move eyes upward or down the other way.

Eventually you'll be comfortable enough with the basic tricks to do some experimenting of your own. There are more stylish mixtures than you could wear in a lifetime. But, for now let's start off with a few sure winners. Here's my suggestions for suits that'll beautifully reshape your specific torso.

Suit your shape

BARRELS

A Chanel-type suit with a contrasting border is a good choice for a short-waisted barrel. The collarless, single-breasted jacket breaks just above the hipline. At this point it safely takes the eye down past the waist. You're left with a great elongating look.

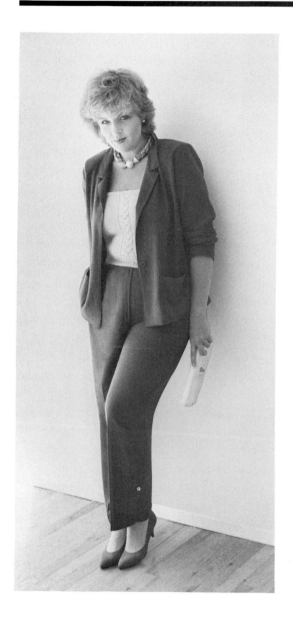

Barrels, of course, are too overpowering around the bustline. Therefore, stay away from jackets with breast pockets, wide lapels, or prominent little insignias. Narrow lapels won't hurt matters, but none at all is best. Unmatched suits must have a solid jacket that's a couple of tones darker than the patterned skirt. For example, a dark blue jacket over a beige and light blue plaid is a combination worth trying.

Slim-fitted skirts will only play up your stomach. I think something with gathers at the hipline or the much-maligned pleated skirt is better for you. Yoke skirts, identified by the V-shaped insert at the waist, work quite well for barrels. They're even more appealing when you have gathers below the broadest section of your tummy. Oh, yes, you barrels can hide a multitude of sins with a slender-legged pantsuit.

BOXES

Your prime objective is to produce at least the facsimile of a waistline. A casual jacket that crisscrosses over your midsection gives a wrap effect. Tie a belt around it and you've accomplished your mission. Another solution would be a fitted, single-breasted jacket that ends three to four inches below your waist. If the neckline is V shape, it helps to visually suggest a waist area.

Skirts should also work on forming a waist, while trying to mold those hips. The dirndl skirt, cut full with a tight waistband, gives you some needed curves. An A-line skirt or a four-piece gore are options too. Gore skirts flare out at the bottom of four panels sewn vertically

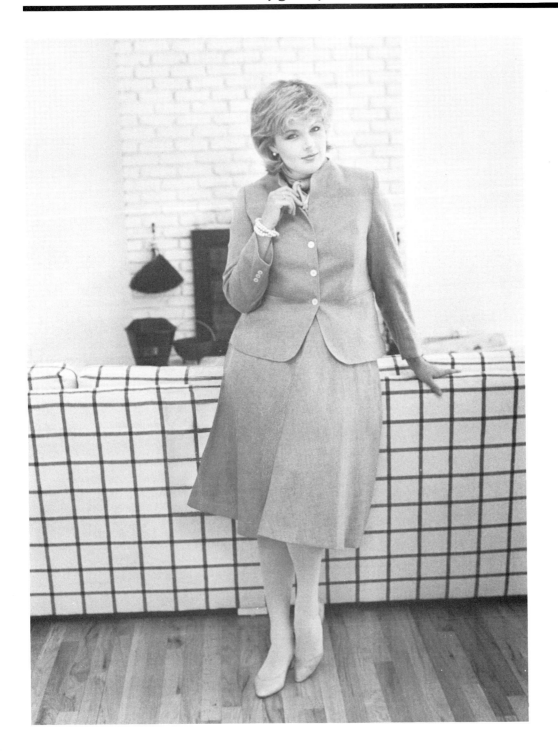

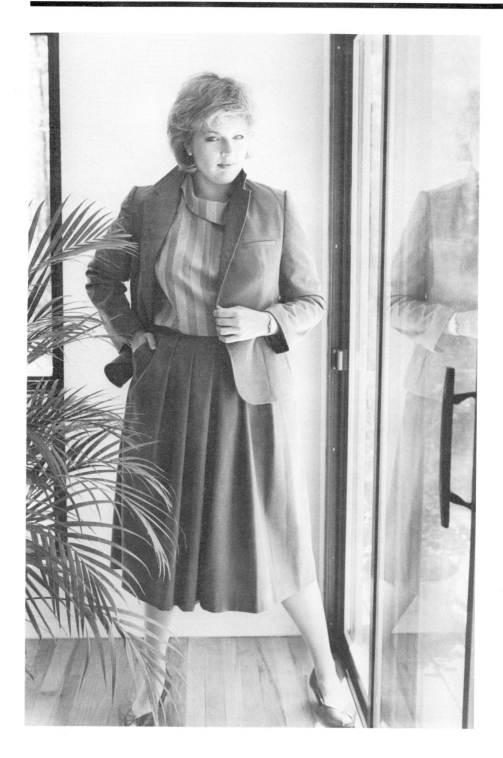

from waist to hemline. The result is an eye-catching but very subtle pattern.

PEARS

All pears want to bring eyes high, away from their bulbous bottoms. At the same time, they should look to broaden typically smaller chests and shoulders. Well, a jacket that stops just above the widest part of the thighs will keep a viewer's gaze up where you prefer it to be. If it's a squarish, unconstructed jacket, the upper torso will seem a lot more substantial. Extended shoulders can be the extra equalizer.

Lower down, try a loosely fitting skirt with soft gathers only in the front. Gathers at the side would automatically bring everybody's attention to your worst features. Actually, a modified A-line skirt might be simpler and more concealing. For a dressier suit, you can check out a knife-pleated skirt topped off by an unbelted tunic jacket. Don't wear any pants or skirts that hug your hips tightly.

FIGURE 8s

Hourglass types thrive in suits that are slightly roomy all over. This gives us just enough material to smooth our extreme curves. Once again, shoulder pads offset big thighs and a sizable caboose. Any boxy jacket without revealing back vents is recommended.

There are quite a few skirts that can compliment a figure 8. A four- or six-piece gore, yokes, front-wrap designs, and the modified A-line are all feasible. By the way, figure 8s are so well proportioned that we benefit from the sameness of fabric and cut of a traditional suit.

Signs of a poor fit

Every aspect of your suit—style, color, pattern, texture—is meaningless if it fits like it was made for your much smaller sister. Don't be one of those women who shrug off bumps, bulges, and stress points by sighing, "Oh well, they all tug at me." Open up a critical eye! Watch out for some common problems and make sure you remedy them before stepping out of the store.

☐ Buttons shouldn't strain against the jacket material while you're trying to close them. Go up to the next size right away!

☐ Pulls rising up in ridges across the back of the jacket means the suit is too small.

☐ Tightness under the arms is another indication of too much size sensitivity and too little stretching room.

☐ Sleeves that expose your naked wrists to the public are absolutely indecent. Either look for some fabric to let down or start searching for a jacket with longer sleeves.

☐ Be sure the waist of the jacket hits you at your natural waistline. If it's too short-waisted, the material around the hips flares out, emphasizing your lower torso. This would be catastrophe for pear-shaped gals.

☐ Collars that stand away or buckle are bad news. You want a collar to lie flat and behave.

☐ Skirts have to allow you to bend and sit without binding, spreading seams, or popping buttons.

☐ You shouldn't have to hold your breath to get your skirt or suit pants zippered up.

☐ Your skirt should be spacious enough for you to walk easily. No tiny, mincing steps, which make you seem awkward.

□ On the other hand, pants or skirts should never bag out in the seat. Too much material is also unsightly.

TOGETHER SEPARATES

Your chances for mixing and matching go beyond the semiformal times that call for a suit. Separates—blouses, sweaters, jeans, slacks, skirts, vests—can be blended into countless outfits just made for looking beautiful while you're hanging out. Each separate you select says something about your fashion savvy, personality, and self-image. Wise choices should combine to give you a youthful air to go along with a seemingly balanced figure. I'd like to provide you with the basic clothing knowledge necessary. The rest is up to you.

Blouses and sweaters

Let's begin the advice at your shoulders and work our way down. If you have a short thick neck, collect sweaters and blouses with scoop or V-shaped openings. Shirts with short collars that stand away from your neck are good, too. They all lengthen the line of your neck by showing a longer stretch of skin. Busty barrels, boxes, or figure 8s also look great in scoops and Vs, but they might be too modest for the open neckline. A shirt with its own limp bow makes a reasonable alternative.

T-shirts and other collarless playthings give you a girlish quality. Too bad thick necks can't handle the uncontoured exposure. In winter, turtlenecks are a mistake because they actually cover too much. Slip on a loose cowl instead, it hints at the possibility of a longer, sen-

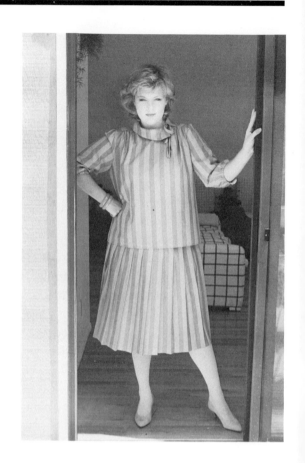

suous neck. Those few women with genuine goose necks can shorten them with jabots, ascots, or Victorian collars.

Most large women are plagued by broad shoulders and heavy arms. For some insane reason we've embraced long, flowing sleeves as the remedy. Bat-winged dolman sleeves, raglans, puffs, and flares are all too wide for husky barrels, figure 8s, and boxes. They only make a massive area more unmissable. Rely on the conventional tailored sleeve and leave the others to the small-topped pears.

When the temperature rises don't try to dress up heavy limbs in elbow-length sleeves. Your arms will come out looking stubby. Either cut back to the half sleeve, or forge forward to a three-quarter length. No sleeve at all would be too revealing.

The overall length of blouses and sweaters is also very important. We've been trying to crawl under a tunic top for years. Generally, they hide nothing and wind up hitting us in the middle of the thighs—the danger zone for all of us, except the barrels. If you insist on salvaging your tunics, shorten them and place a loose belt around the waist. Figure 8s and boxes just might pull it off.

Never purchase really long sweaters! We don't want to become wide shapeless arrows pointing the way to the broadest section of our hips. Pears should take special care in keeping their sweaters at waist level. They can even put on a short, bulky sweater that pulls eyes firmly upward and creates a sense of balance.

Use colors and patterns in your separates the way you did with suits. For instance, our problem pears can do wonders with a dark suit, light sweater, and striped shirt collar showing over the neckline. Barrels can reverse things by wearing a pale pair of pants under a slightly longer dark sweater. Think each outfit through and remember to take the texture of the sweaters into consideration.

Slacks, jeans, and vests

Slacks supposedly tailored for the fuller-figure women have been a thorn in my side since I began modeling. The manufacturers mean well, but many of them can't get their pants together. They think that cutting a leg full all the way down is a blessing. Nonsense! You just get a floppy-legged style with too much material. Other common pants problems are overly wide leg openings, excessive space from crotch to waist, and the never-say-die tightness around the thighs.

Yet now there are some beautiful pants for us on the market. They're usually expensive, but rare commodities seldom come cheaply. Spend your money on pants that are well made, lined, and in style. Don't backslide into the pull-on polyester monstrosities with the presewn creases marring the front.

Jeans are another story. The stores are full of brands that are reasonably priced and do justice to a large frame. In fact, I did nationwide television commercials for a pair that fit me terrifically. However, you have to be able to envision yourself in jeans. It's part of the thinking-young self-image we talked about. Not every woman, big or petite, sees herself as the denim type.

Once you decide to wear jeans, I suggest you try on the stretch denims first. I have both kinds and wind up wearing the stretch constantly, while the others never get out of the closet. Even though the stretch gives somewhat, avoid the extremely tight fit. It might be the rage, but we can't handle it. Go for comfort and a flat smooth lie.

A popular addition to the pants world are the jogging togs. The elastic waist and sweat-shirt fabric are as comfortable as they look. But sweat-pants unmercifully reveal everything. Pears shouldn't even think about them! The rest of you can take a run at them if your body is relatively firm.

Vests are an extra every large woman should investigate. Any old thrift-shop vest personalizes your look while disguising the size of your chest. Both barrels and pears use them for just that purpose. When buying a vest make sure it stops before the hipbone, choose colors that coincide with your outfits, and pick a texture that doesn't rub the other separates the wrong way. Steer clear of the polyester vests in loud prints that go right down to mid-thigh. Ugh!

Footwear facts

Once upon a time, I wore three-inch heels wherever I went. I thought they made me look slimmer, sexier, daintier, longer and more chic. Well, believe me there's nothing worse than seeing a full figure 8 (pear, or box shape) with heavy legs teetering on a pair of spikes. It rates somewhere between clumsy and ridiculous. Thank goodness lower-heeled shoes have come back into my life.

A simple, low pump is the most flattering style for any large woman, no matter how substantial or slim her legs. Short, chunky legs

are particularly wrong for high heels. All you're doing is drawing attention to them. Ankle or T-straps also get people staring at your legs. Colorwise, don't flaunt shoes that contrast too much with any dark-toned hosiery you may wear. And never sink to totally flat shoes, unless you've got long legs attached to slim ankles.

Boots are fine for large women who are smart enough to watch their steps. I get a kick out of cowboy boots. They can be worn with skirts or jeans, and my calves don't wind up being squeezed. If you want to wear a mid-calf type, be sure your hemline meets the top of the boot, to prevent a break in the vertical line of your leg. Short, scrunchy boots are okay on really long, slender legs. Barrels should go right ahead and tuck their jeans into them.

A coat for all seasons

As a rule, keep your coats light and flexible. Thick materials will only add to your general bulk. In autumn, cashmere or a cashmere blend gives you a rich, lean appearance. Women with smaller budgets can get similar results with an enormous variety of wool or wool blends.

Winter presents more of a problem for large women. Quilted coats are difficult for us to wear. If you must have one, don't buy something short or over stuffed. Horizontal seams are a disaster too. Pick an upside-down V pattern that has a slimming, diagonal effect. Vertical lines also fit the bill.

I don't know too many fuller-figure gals who would refuse a fur coat. So, I won't be silly enough to suggest it. But, please show a little discretion. Stick to longer, sleeker coats with a vertical grain. Before putting the fur on try to flatten the pelts, rather than fluff them up. Chubbies and other bushy jackets are obviously a poor investment.

Come spring, be careful to choose coats that cater to your body type. Figure 8s, barrels, and boxes blossom in a straight-A or modified-A shape. Boxes and figure 8s can also flourish in wrap coats that are belted. Capes in water-repellent fabrics do a lovely job of keeping short-waisted barrels and hippy pears out of April showers.

A reminder: We don't wear any raincoats on hot, sunny days. Summer is for bare skin and cool separates.

THE NECESSITY OF ACCESSORIES

Accessories aren't fashion luxuries to save for lavish occasions. They're mainly hard-working jewelry, scarves, and handbags that can make or break your appearance every single day. The lack of accessories often leaves a smashing dress looking dull. Too many extra touches can bury a delicate ensemble. You have to find the items necessary to give your clothes, body, and personality a simple sense of completeness.

What price jewelry?

The smart jewelry isn't measured in carats, ounces, or paper dollars. Never let brilliant luster or glaring price tags blind you. I always dig into the costume-jewelry bins before scanning the satin-covered display cases. I want the pieces that look best on me for the least amount of money. After all, the gist of this book is to be big and beautiful; not narrow and gaudy.

When buying any kind of jewelry, keep your size and proportions in mind. We fuller-figure gals can get away with larger trappings than the skinnies. For example, I'll go for fairly noticeable pearl or gold earrings to offset my substantial head. Anything too small only throws off the balance by comparison. Bold earrings also make a statement about my self-image. I'm tastefully dangling my assertiveness for all to see.

However, even the most liberated ladies should abide by a few prudent rules. Primarily, don't ever buy something without trying it on. Granted, jewelry doesn't bind like a faulty girdle, but it does have to mesh with your features. People with short necks can really appreciate what I mean. One glance in a mirror convinces them never to wear chokers. Another quick appraisal then proves that a long chain clearly adds inches to the line of their throats.

I'm pretty cautious about where I place jewelry, too. There's an old antique watch that I used to wear on a cleavage-length chain. It was a hypnotic timepiece that captured everybody's eye. Finally, I realized that the men around me never got past my chest. I decided to shorten the chain out of modesty and self-defense.

Broaches, stickpins, and cameos can give you similar problems. If an area of your body embarrasses you, don't highlight it with a glittering object. On the other hand, it's a great way to lead a viewer to what you want him to see. Rings cause people to focus on graceful hands. Lots of bracelets enliven long arms with small wrists. And pendulous earrings elongate a wide face.

Dancing scarves

In Baghdad, women suggestively played up the ripest parts of their figures in The Dance Of A Thousand Veils. Today's large gals can still maximize their assets by shifting brightly colored scarves from place to place. It's sort of an exotic fashion dance, but the ripe areas are being hidden this time. The scarves are meant both to deceive and entice.

All large women, except barrels, can begin by draping a long silky scarf around their necks. Let it fall down below your chest and tie a prominent knot. This yanks the eye away from a bulky area. It also complements whatever outfit you have on.

Boxes and figure 8s next remove the scarf to spiral it farther down their bodies. At your waist it becomes a lively substitute for a typical belt. The bright colors mesmerize onlookers and keep them from concentrating elsewhere. It's a dramatic way for a box to invent a waistline.

An extra-large triangular scarf is brought into the dance. You'll recognize it as something popular in the past, which is again fashionable. You can tie it almost anywhere, but I've got my special preference. Shimmy it over your shoulders as a fabulous shawl. Dull dresses or blouses are infused with color, while quite a few upper-torso ills are covered up.

Work freely with scarves, think of uses, and let your dance twirl on.

Find your bag

No outfit is complete without a bag of some kind. We all have our favorites, whether a clutch bag you slip under an arm or an attaché style or the perennial shoulder bag. Just make sure the one you pick isn't too small for your needs and size. A puny purse makes the woman holding it appear that much bigger.

The prime concern about shoulder bags is how far down they hang. If you're beefy in the fanny, shorten the strap so it doesn't hit you too low. A bag by your buns brings attention to that area. However, a barrel is better off with a low-slung bag. It's hard to stare at a big chest when a sizable bag is swaying around the hips.

I think it's foolish to rely on just one bag. Get different styles and colors to go with outfits, moods, evenings, work, *et cetera*. The more bags you have the longer each one will last. Over a period of time it's not any more expensive than buying them one by one.

SEW IT YOURSELF

Many of us, especially ladies living in rural areas, have trouble finding everything we want in the stores. I've always found home sewing a great alternative. You get complete control over the fabrics being used, details of the garment, and lower overall cost. It's a perfect combination of handmade quality and less-than-store-bought prices.

Sewing at home also gives you a chance to tailor the pattern to your exact dimensions. Come to think of it, the clothes my mother sewed for me years ago were the first ones to fit properly. If the idea of making your own outfits appeals to you, don't back away because it sounds difficult. I've asked Ms. Carmen Digilio, master seamstress at Butterick Patterns, to give us some introductory tips for the fuller-figure woman who wants to begin sewing for herself.

Here are her suggestions.

1 *Measure yourself* carefully before shopping for a pattern.

2 Stick to *simple patterns!* Wait until you're more skilled before you get fancy.

3 *Pinfit all patterns* to insure proper fit. This entails pinning the pattern together and carefully trying it on. Have somebody help you. Lightly mark any spots that need adjustments. Never do any cutting before the pinning. You can then make it in muslin after you've made the corrections.

4 *Make adjustments* by the book. First, check for the typical things that need adjustments. Are the bustline, sleeves, waistband, or armholes too tight? If the answer is yes, then cut that pattern section in half. Now, add extra inches at the center of the pattern piece. Otherwise, you'll wind up with a lopsided garment.

Patterns can also be adjusted by moving the bustline up or down. This allows any darts to hit in the correct spot. Make sure that the darts are not above or below the fullest part of the bust. Armholes shouldn't be too high or low, either. Low armholes leave a spread-bat-wing effect.

5 Adapt the *length of the back* to your body.

6 Check your *hemline.* Allow some extra material in the length for tummy bulges up front or fanny rises in the rear. Those chalk measuring sticks are great for marking an even hemline.

7 *Waistbands lined with elastic* are recommended for pants or skirts. They fit more comfortably and don't bind if your weight fluctuates a bit. This doesn't mean omit zippers.

I hope these pointers help you to get through your first, second, or even tenth home-sewn outfit. Read over your body-proportion notes as well. They'll help you choose the correct fabrics and styles for your figure. Everything about your wardrobe should follow a well-planned fashion strategy. After all, nobody is dressed right by accident.

PART THREE

FIGURING THE

NEW YOU—SOON

INTRODUCTION: A BETTER BODY PROGRAM

So far, we've got you thinking, grooming, and dressing like a Big Beauty. I bet you're starting to feel pretty good about yourself. Well, that seems fine to me. But don't expect to look your very best without making some flesh-and-muscle improvements first. There's no substitute for a slightly trimmer, healthier body. Sooner or later, you have to get physical!

Actually, we can use this part of the book to shape up together. I've got to shoot the revealing spring-summer catalogs. Ever since last summer I've been in a tiresome, claustrophobic state. My busy work schedule combines with the cold winds to keep me indoors, inactive, and eating just to break up the days.

What we need is a dynamic, multifaceted approach that will really get us on track in a hurry. My sister's old three-week calorie conservation is a great place to begin. But I'll show you how to update it into a more efficient, varied, and satisfying food plan. Those three weeks will also include regular body-toning recreation and plenty of spine-aligning posture pointers.

You'll get each phase of this "Better Body Program" in separate chapters: "Food In Focus," "The Joys of Fitness," "Posture and Perk." Everything will be broken down into step-by-step instructions. All the important details are unmistakably clear.

Each chapter could qualify as a complete, comprehensive program of it's own.

However, they're meant to be used in an integrated self-help effort. Follow the chapters concurrently so any one of them can reinforce the others. For example, a nutritiously sane way of eating provides you with more energy for the games you play. Conversely, an invigorating workout cuts down your appetite. Correct posture leaves you pain free for sports. And certain physical activities return the favor by strengthening the back muscles.

The real beauty of my program is how often you attain meaningful, short-range goals. I personally foresee losing at least the equivalent of a five-pound bag of sugar. (Doesn't that sound like a fairly big burden to get off your body in just three weeks!) My figure should also be noticeably firmer; my movements will appear more graceful. I'll also be in closer touch with my body.

I know the popular fad diets promise you larger weight losses. Too bad it's usually water and valuable muscle tissue being shed instead of fat. Rigid exercising regimens order you to whip yourself into rock-hard shape. In truth, you usually wind up only sore, frustrated, or injured. None of these blitz attacks can fit into the scheme of your life for long. When the struggle is over you immediately put the pounds back on, while your body plumps out again to the old status quo.

My system works steadily to modify your current habits. There's a natural flexibility purposely retained in the suggestions. Room is allotted for the inevitable ups and downs, desires, and special occasions we all face. After the three weeks are up, you should find the next three weeks even easier to get through. Hopefully, you'll be creating better behavior patterns that will last for years to come.

CHAPTER EIGHT

FOOD IN FOCUS

Just about every large woman I know has a similar blind spot. Wait, don't tell me how great your eyesight is! Even you ladies with twenty/twenty vision seem to have trouble seeing the way you relate to food. Our eating habits often become obscured into one big blur. The amount of food we consume is forever getting overlooked. Most of us go so far as to lose sight altogether of the real reasons for eating.

Happily, I only suffer from this malady during my autumn blahs. For nine months a year, I have the whys and what-to-dos of eating in sharp focus. When I'm on my shape-up program or maintenance (explained in "Beyond the New You—Later") food is seen primarily as a source of nourishment. That doesn't mean I give up the tastes of mouth-watering delicacies. I merely cut down on my overall calorie intake. Then, I try limiting myself to the "quality calories" that have true nutritional value.

The transition to my wiser style of eating begins, appropriately, by opening your eyes. Here you attempt to closely observe your personal idiosyncrasies. At first, you'll be looking mostly for mistakes. This is a surface and soul-searching preparation for the positive three-week food plan ahead. The idea is to be totally aware of all the little things you feel and do that are responsible for blowing you up.

By the way, saying you recognize a bad habit is not enough. You usually just hear it for a second and then it's gone. In my program even the wrong turns get spelled out. In other words, every false step is written down in an "eating diary." Later on, when you're following my better way, all the right moves you make get recorded in the same daily ledger.

Writing bad habits

Examining your bad habits doesn't take quite as long as establishing good ones. I rev up for my food plan by zeroing in on the four previous days. This gives me several kinds of situations to analyze. The meals, moods, and details of each day are recent enough to remember well. But since they've already happened, I can't consciously clean up my act as I go along. Sugar coating the facts is the last thing we should do at this point!

My decision to get back to healthy eating came in late November. Therefore, the abuses of Thanksgiving gluttony were still weighing heavy on my body and mind. The time to be scrutinized ran from before the big holiday through the dreaded day after. I took the eating events of each day as a separate entity. Unlike the food plan to come, no progress tallies were carried over to the next day. Surprisingly, my scribblings revealed that turkey dinner (with all the trimmings) was not the worst of my problems.

Setting up your diary to chart these bad habits is relatively simple. The pages are arranged like menus of *what you ate*. Entries cover everything from morning's first sips of coffee to evening's final bites. In front of each item is the estimated *amount consumed* in

ounces, teaspoons, pieces, *et cetera*. Where the costs of the food is usually listed on a menu we've placed the approximate *calorie count*. I advise buying a pocket-sized calorie book for quick-figuring accuracy.

A tabulation of your calories doesn't show exactly what brought about the damages. You should note *where you ate* different parts of the day's fare. Eating in kitchens, bedrooms, offices, or cars indicates specific kinds of trouble. The *time you ate* each thing, *who was with you*, and *your mood* at every sitting helps to flesh out the picture even more. Finally, rate your *degree of hunger* at the moment each morsel passed through your lips. Your comments should range from "not hungry" to "ravenous."

Don't get upset by the one time you chomped donuts on the way to work. However, gooey second breakfasts in the car for two mornings straight is a four-alarm warning. You're showing evidence of several fattening habits. The solution is to see them for what they are and then make the proper changes. Perhaps a look at my four "bad" days will make your job a little easier. Each day in the diary is followed by my own analysis of the information recorded.

Ann's big bad days

Day 1, Tuesday

food eaten	*calories*

Breakfast (8:30 A.M.), at home in T.V. room, alone, moderately hungry

2-egg swiss-cheese (2 ounces) omelet in 1 tablespoon butter	500

8 ounces orange juice	100
poppy-seed bagel	300
2 tablespoons cream cheese	106
cappuccino with 4 ounces whole milk	83
2 teaspoons sugar	36
total:	1,125

Lunch (12 noon), in the den at desk, alone, agitated, not hungry

meatball hero (from Angelo's at the corner)	500
6½ ounce bag potato chips	1014
12 ounce can cola	144
brownie	141
total:	1,799

Snack 4 P.M.), in T.V. room, alone, somewhat bored, not hungry

cookies (20 cream filled)	800
pint whole milk	232
total:	1,032

Nap (4:30 P.M.)

Drinks (7:30 P.M.), living room, with a few friends, elated, sort of hungry

2 (12 ounces) glasses Beaujolais wine	288
1¼ ounce blue cheese	131
1 ounce Camembert cheese	86
1 ounce cheddar cheese	113
10 crackers	220
total:	838

Dinner (9 P.M.), restaurant, with same friends, psyched up, thinking food

3 glasses (16 ounces) red wine	336
pâté de campagne	250
popover	90
2 teaspoons butter	70
salad (mixed greens) and blue-cheese dressing	292
baked potato with 2 ounces sour cream and 1 ounce butter	256
16 ounce sirloin steak (rare)	1,848
sautéed onions	145
cheesecake (one average piece)	300
espresso	1
anisette	102
total:	3,690

Total calories for the day:	8,484

ANALYSIS: DAY 1, TUESDAY

I know an eight-thousand-calorie day sounds awfully excessive. Some of you might be thinking that it's absolutely absurd. "I would never go that crazy!" you say. Well, I think it's run-of-the-mill for plenty of people, especially large women who aren't aware of their bad habits. I didn't even go for any hot-fudge sundaes, candy bars, eclairs, or mid-morning snacks.

Yet, the number of calories ingested was more than three times what I might be allowed on maintenance. Also, the quantity of food consumed surprised me. I never expected the list to be so long. Writing things down suddenly made the eating loom larger and the lack of exercise seem more obvious. Work-at-home days had recently become very hazy in retrospect.

A percentage of that haziness translated into bad eating habits. Breakfast blended into the drone of the television. I never really concentrated on what I was eating. I whipped up a meal to accompany a whole hour's worth of talk shows, rather than cooking lightly to coincide with a "moderate" hunger. Those heavy omelets would've never made it into the buttered frying pan if I had intended to sit at the dining-room table.

Lunch also got inadvertently blown out of proportion. It was due to a combination of laziness, the wrong frame of mind, and another case of eating with distractions. I originally went for a morning walk to get some exercise. Instead, I got as far as Angelo's at the corner of my block. I thought, why take time to fix up a measly little lunch when I can *buy* a two-fisted feast? And I soothed my conscience by planning to eat only half the stuff at noon, while saving the rest for a late-afternoon snack.

That's obviously not the way it turned out. The whole idea of buying lunch was to give me more time to work on this book. So I sprawled my goodies out on the desk and began checking material. Read and bite, read and sip, cross out a line and two bites. After three pages I was over halfway through the hero, soda, and chips.

On the fifth page I really got stuck. An awkward section was driving me cuckoo. I could feel myself getting impatient, then plain agitated. Next thing I knew, every scrap was history except the brownie. One more lame shot at the passage in front of me and I devoured the brownie on spite.

My major sin was making overeating so easy. Store-cooked lunches take all the effort out of piling up calories. Once the food was bought, half of everything should have been wrapped in tinfoil and shut away. After all,

those distractions can be made to work two ways. They can also prevent you from making a long trek to the kitchen in search of more food. Besides, the extra time it takes to get there gives you an opportunity to change your mind.

The snack at four was a matter of predetermination. I decided from the moment I woke up that some tasty reward was going to be waiting for me when the work was done. Earlier, it appeared that half the booty from Angelo's was earmarked for this purpose. Those twenty cream-filled cookies and milk were just a last-minute substitution.

In the future, I'll make a point of not setting myself up for unwanted calories. I wasn't hungry! I was sort of bored and then tired from the constant eating. My nap didn't leave me refreshed, and nothing I ate got burned off. Once the body program begins I'll use this part of the day for recreation. It can be my reward and a way to drop calories, too.

Having friends over got me out of my funk. I was happy and naturally wanted to reinforce that high with a bit of wine. Sometimes I forget how fattening alcoholic drinks can be. Sweet wines tend to have more calories per ounce than the dryer ones. Cheese and crackers can also run up more calories than people give them credit for.

In fact, the crackers (like the soda, cookies, brownie, *et cetera*) I ate had a lot of hidden empty calories. A cracker's dextrose and maltose are forms of processed sugar, which have no nutritional value. Whole-grain bread would have been a lot more nutritious and filling. Who knows, I might have eaten less. As it is, the average American (forget about the average fuller-figure nibbler) packs away about 120 pounds of processed sugar a year.

Finally, we come to that extravagant restaurant dinner. I love ordering fine meals! Yet, on occasion, my zeal for haute cuisine overshadows my better judgment. There's simply no chance for a load of rich dishes to be properly digested so close to bedtime.

I should have skipped the pâté, popover and butter, blue-cheese dressing, and two glasses of wine. An eight-ounce steak would have been more than sufficient and the cheesecake could have been shared with a friend. At that hour, even the anisette was overkill when one calorie of espresso tops off a meal just elegantly. Remember, late-night calories are more likely to be retained by your body.

ANN'S BIG BAD DAYS

Day 2, Wednesday

food eaten	calories

Breakfast (7:30 A.M.), while getting dressed, rushed, moderately hungry

8 ounces apple cider	112
English muffin	140
2 teaspoons butter	66
strawberry preserves	78
total:	396

Snack (9:00 A.M.), arrive studio, preparing, hassled, not hungry

coffee with whole milk and sugar	40
one long piece of strudel	200
total:	240

Lunch (12 noon), restaurant, with mag. editor, anxious, not hungry

2 bloody marys	192
eggs benedict	550
salad with vinaigrette dressing	100
fruit compote (in syrup)	250
coffee with whole milk and sugar	40
total:	1,132

Shooting 3:00 P.M.–5:00 P.M.

Snack (5:45 P.M.), in kitchen, alone, weary, slightly hungry

8 ounces Beaujolais wine	168
leftover cheese and crackers	about 400
total:	568

Dinner (8 P.M.), in dining room, one friend, mellow, slightly hungry

8 ounces Gewürztraminer (fruity, white) wine	196
sautéed pork chops (12 ounces)	1,290
mashed potatoes	188
gravy	205
canned peas and carrots	104
1/2 pint of chocolate ice cream	375
3 tablespoons butterscotch topping	165
1 ounce peanuts	180
total:	2,703
Total calories for the day:	5,039

ANALYSIS; DAY 2, WEDNESDAY

This was one of my on-the-move workdays. Up early! Two shootings and lunch with a women's-magazine editor on the agenda. My breakfast was also eaten while in motion. It was filling, tasty, and maybe a little too heavy on empty calories. Yet, in my mind, it was eaten too rush-rush to count as an official breakfast. So, when strudel and coffee was offered at the studio, I felt entitled to partake.

Business lunches are murder for anybody remotely concerned with healthy eating. I walked into the restaurant feeling a tad nervous and anxious to sound good. Naturally, I couldn't let the editor drink alone. Wham! Almost two hundred calories guzzled before the menu arrives. Maybe, I should've kept her company with mineral water or a white-wine spritzer instead.

Honestly, I wasn't the least bit hungry at lunchtime. If I were out on my own, I might not have eaten much at all. But, I couldn't refuse to order big at the editor's "favorite restaurant." It's always *somebody's* favorite restaurant. I thought I was being fairly good by getting the salad, eggs, and fruit. I just forgot to consider the Benedict's rich sauce and the compote's fattening syrup.

Preparing a sizable dinner when you're tired is like playing into the calorie devil's hands. Your resistance is low, food is all around you, and exhaustion is so easy to confuse with hunger. I found it especially easy to squeeze in an unnecessary snack because I had all those cheese remnants lying around from the day before. I convinced myself that eating them up was the same as cleaning out the refrigerator.

Hallelujah! Dinner was finally eaten in the right place—sitting attentively at the dining-room table. But there were still a couple of

killer mistakes. Number one, I overestimated the amount of food necessary to satisfy two people. There was easily enough pork, potatoes, and everything else to stuff four hungry adults. On more alert days I would take the time to measure portions.

My second blunder was to serve all this food family style. Seeing platters stacked high with edibles seems to act as a challenge to hearty eaters. Let's face it, most of us are trained to gobble down whatever is put in front of our eyes. So we both went a little wild and only left a few drops over. Of course, I stuck the survivors into the fridge for later pickings.

Oh, yes, Tuesday and Wednesday were both lopsided with fats. A majority of the foods listed seem to contain an inordinate amount. Just look at all the cheeses, eggs, butter, whole milk, meats, cakes, crackers, ice cream. It's almost like skipping the middle man and packing the fat right on to my body.

DAY 3, THURSDAY, THANKSGIVING

Now, a little change in procedure here. The food, calories, and events on Thanksgiving, not to mention the day after, got somewhat out of hand. In fact, more things went down (food-wise) than the diary is capable of reporting. So, for the sake of comprehension and expediency, I'll just intermingle the diary with the analysis. This leaves us with an introspective summary of the damage.

Breakfast was consciously kept to a minimum. I only had cappuccino with half of a toasted bagel and butter. I was building up an excuse for going hog-wild later. This breakfast was an attempt to undercut guilt in advance. You know, "I'm saving myself for the Big Meal."

I arrived early at my brother's and sister-in-law's house to help set things up. I was also the first one to sample the goodies each member of the family promised to bring. By two o'clock all offerings had been transferred to serving plates and personally "checked in." Just in time for predinner drinks and hors d'oeuvres.

Thanksgiving always seems to be accompanied by a string of football games. Drinks and hors d'oeuvres became a reflection of what was going on in the games. I cut back and forth around the living room tackling every relative's dish. After each mouthful was downed, I made a point of passing a few words of appreciation in the right direction.

"Ruth, this Brie wheel you baked in a crust is utterly delicious," I yelled over the noise of the crowd. Ruth nodded, took a bite of Lucille's liver pâté, and gave her a similar compliment. A few daiquiris later, I had given every cheese, quiche, and vegetable concoction its well-deserved pat on the back. In truth, it was all delicious. But the complimenting allows you to convince yourself that you're only stuffing it down to be polite.

At six o'clock the Big Meal was upon us. I wasn't hungry until I sat down at the dining-room table. The ravenous vibrations sent out by twelve people in the holiday spirit went right to my stomach. An enormous turkey, mounds of stuffing, golden-crisp potatoes, home-baked raisin bread, creamed onions, mixed vegetables, my cranberry conserve, and pumpkin and pecan pies all tempted me at once. I grabbed for them in pairs, never allowing my plate to be totally full or empty.

Eating two things at a time makes it impossible to keep track of how much food is being consumed. There's something more definite and final about filling up one plate with a bit of each dish. You feel more compelled to finish what's in front of you and push back from the table. Obviously, putting together complete plates of food catches the attention of the people around you. A third complete plate is unavoidable.

DAY 4, FRIDAY, THE DAY AFTER

A slight confession—I look forward to this day more than Thanksgiving itself. I even planned to stay over at my brother's house. Oh, that morning-after turkey sandwich! I wouldn't have missed it for the world.

9:30 A.M. turkey piled high (white and dark meat)
2 pieces of rye toast
bacon, lettuce, and tomato
gobs of mayonnaise
2 8-ounce glasses of whole milk
half a plate of cold stuffing

The remainder of the day was spent nibbling and talking. I hovered in and around the kitchen being "sociable." Demurely, I refused a formal lunch platter just before noon. "Nah, I'll just pick on a few scraps," I shrugged. What could've been better? Martyr and mammoth eater all in one breath.

I made my way home that evening with a goodie basket. "Here's tomorrow's supper for you," my sister-in-law said at the door. "En-joy!" I certainly did that. Every morsel was eaten on the ride home. It's hard to notice the food going when one hand is on the wheel and your eyes are on the road.

In essence, I did a stretching act with Thanksgiving. I managed to take one holiday meal and extend it into a two-day binge. In my mind it was okay—acceptable. I'm sup-posed to celebrate and join the feast. But even the holiday "spirit" has a rough time support-ing about thirty thousand calories over forty-eight hours. I don't want Christmas to be a carbon copy.

Food for thought

Nobody leaps directly from a heavy binge into an enlightened eating routine. Heck, my first reaction was to go on a semistarvation diet. I woke up the next morning thinking, "If I can just skip a meal or two a day, everything will balance out real fast." It's the kind of panicky response that even the most knowledgeable women have. The old grab-the-bull-by-the-horns mentality.

Once I calmed down, the reasoning behind the stop-eating attack sort of fell apart. I real-ized that my stomach was stretched out of shape right then. The hunger pangs from going cold turkey (no Thanksgiving pun in-tended) would surely prompt another round of stuffing myself. Besides, deliberately skip-ping meals shifts your body's metabolism into a much lower gear. I'd be losing weight more slowly by burning up calories at a snail's pace.

No, I couldn't afford to rush into a whole new set of problems. I would take the weekend to get priorities straight in my head. A successful food plan has to cope with the mistakes exposed during the "bad days." It's the only way to lose weight—while reintro-ducing myself to a healthier approach to eat-ing. Monday would be soon enough to start the three-week march to a trimmer me.

Counting calories

Obviously, when I must go on a food plan, I'm not going to drop pounds by rolling up more than five thousand calories on every flip of a diary page. There's just so much your body can burn away in a twenty-four-hour period. So, I've decided to put a fifteen-hundred-calorie limit on my intake. I know many "stricter" diets insist that you stay under eight hundred calories a day. But it's too big an adjustment for me to make after my escapades. I might never be ready for that kind of restriction.

However, a daily maximum of fifteen hun-dred calories permits me to comfortably reach my reducing goal for the program. I'll be con-suming about seven hundred to one thousand calories a day *below* the amount I require to maintain my weight. (Of course, maintenance needs vary according to your size, age, ac-tivity level, *et cetera*.) By the end of each week, my calorie deficit should be great enough to guarantee about a two-pound loss. After three weeks, my five-pound target seems to be the least I can expect.

Naturally, there will be days when I manage to eat a bit less than the fifteen hundred calories allowed. Those calories shouldn't get lost in the shuffle. I deserve a little extra credit for them. I don't mean just a few gushy words of praise. I'm talking about the type of credit you can spend later on.

Say the diary shows that I've ingested only thirteen hundred calories on a Monday. I subtract the thirteen hundred from the fifteen hundred calories considered acceptable. My two hundred calories left over are placed on a slip of paper. That slip is then deposited into a "savings envelope" taped to the back cover of my diary. During the week, I'm permitted to add any part of what's in the envelope to the fifteen-hundred-calorie ceiling of a particular day. Or else, if a festive weekend is coming up, I can wait and just blow the whole savings at once.

This credit system was my sister Ruth's innovation. In fact, most of the food plan is a synthesis of food-control ideas I've picked up from various sources over the years. They meld into a system that makes each component work better together than they each did alone. For instance, I've modified Ruth's suggestion somewhat. In my plan you can't carry any credit over to the next week. And there are elements in the food plan that make huge calorie days awfully difficult to cram in.

Shrinking meals

One way to prevent calorie sprees is to change the whole concept of meals. Let's shrink these multicourse productions that encourage you to eat as much as possible three times a day. All they do is stretch your stomach and eating capacity beyond controllable bounds. Large meals also help to manufacture more insulin, which promotes the conversion of sugars and complex carbohydrates into fats.

Simply, I intend to *eat smaller amounts* of food at each sitting. Both the size of the portions and the number of courses served will be decreased. This should cause my tummy to contract. In a short while, I'll reach the point where soup-to-nuts suppers become prohibitively uncomfortable.

My other ploy is to *eat more often*. That's right! Tiny meals on a frequent basis have almost the opposite effect of skipping eating. Your metabolism hums along at a torrid rate evaporating the pockets of calories in its path. *Five or six "minimeals" daily* should also be just about right for warding off the hunger that makes empty-calorie snacks so inviting.

Actually, there won't be snacks of any description in my food plan. Whatever you choose to eat must be seen as a minimeal. When we label something a "snack" there's a tendency to negate the need for calorie control or top nutritional value. Snacks are so often down graded to nothing more than casually munching candy or some other kind of junk food. That's letting them off much too easily.

Exchanging foods

Allotting myself a practical amount of calories per diem is a smart initial move. My minimeal format appears to be a wise method for handling hunger and metabolic concerns. But the genius of the food plan hinges on how I actually spend those precious fifteen hundred calories. I could never tolerate an inflexible, morning-to-night diet menu. That would get too boring to sustain for any length of time. So I've always depended on a unique food system that offers a balanced selection of many *interchangeable* items.

Basically, we're talking about Food Exchange Lists developed by a joint committee of the American Dietetic Association, the American Diabetes Association, and the United States Public Health Service. These lists were created to help you get the most out of a limited number of calories. You're supposed to choose your day's minimeals from five different "food groups": *Milk, Vegetable, Fruit, Bread*, and *Meat*. A sixth group of *Fats* should be avoided (as should alcohol) because of its extremely high concentration of calories.

Every single one of the groups contains a homogeneous listing of foods in varying quantities. For example, the Meat Group includes chicken (1 ounce), cold cuts (1 slice), tuna (¼ cup) and shrimp (3–5 medium size). I know their individual amounts seem rather far apart or random. Yet, every item on a particular list is considered to be an equal "unit" for our purposes.

What allows these irregular units to claim equality? That's the key to the entire exchange process. Primarily, the answer has to do with the three calorie-carrying nutrients. Each list is worked out so all of its items are *about* the same in carbohydrate, protein, and fat content. Therefore, every item on a list is relatively equal in calories and plausibly *interchangeable* in a calorie-counting food plan.

As you'll see, making lists up by nutrient content can sometimes make a few strange

Food exchange lists

LIST 1: MILK GROUP

One unit contains approximately 85 calories, 12 grams of carbohydrates, 8 grams of protein, under 1 gram fat.

buttermilk	1	cup
partially skimmed milk	¾	cup
skim milk	1	cup
ice milk	⅓	cup
cottage cheese, creamed	⅓	cup
yogurt, fruit and flavored	½	cup
yogurt, plain (skim milk)	1	cup

LIST 2: VEGETABLE GROUP

One unit contains about 25 calories, 5 grams of carbohydrates, 2 grams protein, under 1 gram fat. Size of all unit servings is ½ cup, cooked.

asparagus	okra
broccoli	onions
brussels sprouts	peppers
cabbage	radishes
carrots	spinach
cauliflower	squash
celery	string beans
cucumbers	tomatoes
eggplant	turnip greens
grains (in general)	turnips
mushrooms	

LIST 3: FRUIT GROUP

One unit contains about 40 calories, 10 grams of carbohydrates, protein and fat negligible. Fruits may be fresh, dried, cooked, canned, or frozen, so long as absolutely no sugar is ever added.

apple	small
apple juice or cider	2 ounces
applesauce	1/2 cup
apricots	2 medium
apricots (dried)	4 halves
banana	1/2 small
blackberries	1 cup
blueberries	2/3 cup
1/4 cantaloupe	6-inch diameter
cherries	10 large
dates	2
fig (dried)	1 small
figs (fresh)	2 large
grapefruit	1/2 small
grapefruit juice	1/2 cup
grape juice	1/4 cup
grapes	12
honeydew melon	1/8 melon
mango	1/2 small
orange	1 small
orange juice	1/2 cup
papaya	1/3 medium
peach	1 medium
pear	1 small
pineapple	1/2 cup (pieces)
pineapple juice	1/3 cup
plums	2 medium
prunes (dried)	2 medium
raspberries	1 cup
strawberries	1 cup
tangerine	1
watermelon	1 cup (pieces)

LIST 4: BREAD GROUP

One unit contains about 70 calories, 15 grams of carbohydrates, 2 grams of protein, fat negligible.

most bread	1 slice
biscuit roll	1 2-inch diameter
cornbread	1 1 1/2-inch cube
muffin	1 2-inch diameter
cereal, cooked	1/2 cup
cereal, flaked and puffed types	3/4 cup
rice and grits cooked	1/2 cup
macaroni and other pastas cooked	1/2 cup
crackers, graham	2 2 1/2-inch square
crackers, oyster	20
crackers, round thins	6
crackers, saltines	5 2-inch square
crackers, soda	3 2 1/2-inch square
flour	2 1/2 tablespoons
baked beans (no pork)	1/4 cup
beans (dried) and peas (cooked)	1/2 cup
corn	1/3 cup
parsnips	2/3 cup
popcorn (without butter)	1 cup
potato	1 small
sweet potatoes or yams	1/4 cup

LIST 5: MEAT GROUP

One unit contains about 75 calories, carbohydrates negligible, 7 grams of protein, 5 grams of fat. If the meat is cut very lean, it will have less fat and, thus, less calories.

meat and poultry: beef, game, lamb, liver, pork, chicken (no visible fat present)	1 ounce
cold cuts	1 slice, 4½ x 1/8-inch
eggs	1
fresh fish: bass, cod, flounder, haddock, halibut, mackerel, salmon	1 ounce
crab, lobster, salmon (canned), tuna	¼ cup, loosely packed
clams, oysters, scallops, shrimps	3-5 medium
peanut butter	1 tablespoon
cheeses: (American, cheddar, swiss, etc.)	1 slice, 4x4x1/8-inch or 1-inch cube or 1 ounce

LIST 6: FAT GROUP

One unit contains about 45 calories, carbohydrates and protein negligible, 5 grams of fat. Try to avoid this group.

1/8 avocado	4-inch diameter
bacon (crisp)	1 slice
butter or margarine	1 teaspoon
cream (heavy)	1 tablespoon
cream (light)	2 tablespoons
cream cheese	1 tablespoon
french dressing	1 tablespoon
mayonnaise	1 teaspoon
nuts	6 small
oil or cooking fat	1 teaspoon
olives	5 small

EXTRA LIST: FREE FOODS.

Unlimited amounts of units are allowed. These foods contain a negligible number of calories.

bouillon (fat free)	mustard
broth, clear	pickle, dill (unsweetened)
coffee (black)	rhubarb (unsweetened)
cranberries (unsweetened)	soy sauce
gelatin (unsweetened)	spices (assorted)
herbs (all kinds)	tea (no milk or sugar)
lemon	vinegar

bedfellows. Take a look at the Bread Group. Besides bread, there are things like potatoes, baked beans, cereal, and corn. A high carbohydrate reading keeps potatoes and corn off the Vegetable Group list. In fact, it's the level of the carbohydrates that distinguishes every item on the Bread Group list.

The number of units you're allowed to take daily from each list is determined by your calorie ceiling. A fifteen-hundred-calorie maximum leaves room for a filling, wide variety of foods. You can eat your allotted units in whatever order or combination you prefer. Some items from a certain list might not appeal to your taste buds. Fine. Just ignore them. Other favorites can be chosen continously in their place.

Here's what you're entitled to eat every day on a *fifteen-hundred-calorie plan:* Milk Group—two units; Vegetable Group—four units; Fruit Group—three units; Bread Group—six units; Meat Group—seven units. If you must have items from the Fat Group, no more than two or three units are ever condoned. Of course, days with no Fat Group selections are the ideal.

Wait one second! I've got a great bonus for us, too. There's a wonderful seventh list we can go to at any time. The "Free Foods" list has no restrictions or unit limitations. It's an assortment of get-through-the-day essentials that have very few—if any—calories. I try to use the free foods to perk up my meals or take the place of a quick high-calorie snack.

You should also note that I haven't added any special "diet" foods, mixes, or powders to the lists. This is just one of many suggestions by Research Nutritionist Sumita Basu

Roy, formerly with St. Luke's-Roosevelt Hospital Obesity Research Center in New York. Dr. Basu Roy, my food-plan adviser, reminds me that the aim of our program is to recondition eating habits and to adopt a normal, nutritionally sound approach to food. It's obvious to her that we can't do this by turning constantly to chemical substitutes for sustenance. She warns us that the long-term effects of frequent use of artificial diet foods are unknown. And some diet foods only reduce salt content and body water without cutting down calories or our fat stores.

However, let me ease your mind a bit about eating the wrong foods. Then I can give you the complete, highly preferred Food Exchange Lists with a clear conscience. THERE ARE NO ABSOLUTELY FORBIDDEN FOODS! A piece of milk chocolate, an ice cream soda, or a napoleon aren't recommended. But, if you eat one of them, it doesn't mean the food plan is ruined. You simply must try to compensate by consuming less calories somewhere else. Or maybe you'll find enough credit in your savings envelope to cover it by the end of the week.

ON THE FOOD PLAN

On Monday, I'm ready to get going. My overall preparation is just about complete. I feel the sensational eagerness that always comes with starting another shape-up cycle. Yet I want to check out a few final points before throwing myself into the food plan, the one part of the program that demands constant monitoring.

In fact, keeping tabs on what I eat is my first

consideration. I have to take on a whole fresh approach to my diary. Unlike the "bad days," the entries should be totally current—recording things as they happen. This means carrying a purse-size book with me all the time. I'll try to make the presence of the written word act as an unshakable conscience.

The layout of each diary page must also change to fit its positive new purpose. Forget about capturing the mood of the moment, the scene of the crime, or the various accomplices that led you astray. Concentrate only on the bookkeeping necessary to document your progress. I expect to see a long, time-staggered list of minimeals running top to bottom. Next to every serving should be the exchange units they represent and the calories involved. Daily calorie surpluses are marked on the page before being deposited into the savings envelope.

Hunger ratings are no longer required, either. I'm already aware of how often I've stuffed myself without really being hungry. Now I have to internalize the basic differences between hunger and appetite. I'll make an effort to separate *true hunger* signals—feelings of emptiness, headaches, irritability—from the less demanding desire for a pleasing taste. You have to know that appetite is more pampering than necessity.

Another thing I've learned over the years is caution. I always make sure to speak with my doctor about any major changes in my diet. I don't want a deficiency or allergy problem brought on by a "special" health condition that might have developed. Besides, the food plan and your initiative will usually elicit a very positive response. And there's nothing

like the unqualified enthusiasm of a doctor to start you off with confidence.

All right, this is it! The shape-up program—food plan in particular—is officially under way. I won't swamp you with a complete account of all twenty-one days. Instead, I'll open up two pages the first week, one the second week, and then the final day for your edification. You should find them a more-than-adequate example of how the diary and food plan work.

Each of these chosen days will be followed by a brief analysis. You'll also get a general progress report at the end of every week. I'll only allow you to jump on the scale for week-closing pick-me-ups. In future cycles, a quick weigh-in and a final weigh-out should be enough.

ANN'S OH-SO-GOOD DAYS

Monday, Week 1

Units allowed: 2 Milk, 4 Vegetable, 3 Fruit, 6 Bread, 7 Meat, 3 Fat
Calories allowed: 1,500

time	food eaten	calories
7:15 A.M.	8 ounces water on rising	
7:30 A.M.	6 ounces apple cider (2½ Fruit)	100
8:15 A.M.	4 ounces skim milk in decaffeinated cappuccino (½ Milk)	43
	1 slice bran toast (1 Bread)	70
	2 teaspoons butter (2 Fat)	90
9:05 A.M.	12 ounces water and vitamins	

11:00 A.M.	8 ounces chicken bouillon (Free)	
1:30 P.M.	1 tablespoon peanut butter (1 Meat)	75
	2 slices bran toast (2 Bread)	140
	8 ounces skim milk (1 Milk)	85
3:10 P.M.	8 ounces seltzer with lime (Free)	
4:05 P.M.	1 hard-boiled egg (1 Meat)	75
	6 ounces tomato juice (1½ Vegetable)	38
6:10 P.M.	½ unsweetened dill pickle (Free)	
7:30 P.M.	8 ounces water before meal	
	5 ounces skinless chicken in vinegar (5 Meat)	300
	1 cup cooked brown rice (2 Bread)	140
	1 cup steamed carrots (2 Vegetable)	50
9:00 P.M.	1 cup popcorn, no butter (1 Bread)	70
10:10 P.M.	1 cup chamomile tea (Free)	
11:00 P.M.	12 ounces water before bed	

total: 1,276
deposit: 224

Units eaten: 1½ Milk, 3½ Vegetable, 2½ Fruit, 6 Bread, 7 Meat, 2 Fat

ANALYSIS, MONDAY, WEEK 1

I'm extremely pleased with the first day of the program. The food plan took off with a 224-calorie deposit for my savings envelope, and I've already started to ease into the ex-ercising routine. I know flying starts come easy, but they're great for the ego. I'm sort of feeling lighter right now (a common illusion) and counting on a three-pound loss by the end of the week.

You might have noticed a couple of extra features in the diary. I wrote the amount of calories and exchange units allowed at the top of the page. They serve as not-so-subtle reminders of my limits every time I go to write something down. A total of the units eaten that day has been inserted at the bottom. This way I can tell at a glance whether I've stayed within the bounds of the plan.

Perhaps the most difficult adjustment was getting into the frequent, minimeal pattern. A few months of eating three feasts a day can spoil you. I had to do a lot of talking to myself, especially before a meal. For instance, at the early evening meal I took a little more time in the preparation. I weighed my portion of chicken carefully prior to marinating and made sure I had no more than one cup of cooked rice.

In the beginning, it's important to get into the habit of weighing portions. A letter scale will do just fine. After a short while, you'll be able to estimate the equivalent of a unit at a glance. Minimizing your courses also takes a bit more thought. I found eating all minimeals at the dining-room table to be a big help in sharpening my concentration.

There were other tricks of the weight-losing trade that contributed to my stellar start. The five units of skinless chicken were quite a few calories below what you might expect. Why? Well, most of the usually invisible fat in chicken is concealed under the skin. If you remove that skin, the fatty calories just go with it.

Water also got me flowing in the right direction. I've decided to drink water (or some other Free Food beverage, like seltzer) whenever I expect to feel hungry. For instance, eight pure ounces before the evening meal fills you up a little—undercutting your desire to gluttonize. Water manages to flush away impurities in your system, combat flu, and help your skin tone, as well. What's more, I often mistake thirst for hunger. So I'll just drink first and play it safe.

At night I was superb! At first I cooked up too much popcorn. But I only took my solitary cupful and threw the rest away. Leftovers like that can get you in trouble. Next time I'll be careful about the amount I prepare. And if I pop it in the microwave, no oil will be needed.

After the nine-o'clock popcorn, I restricted myself to Free liquids. Therefore, I went to sleep without difficult-to-digest foods or a load of calories wedged in my stomach. I slept better and didn't wake up a half pound heavier.

Ann's oh-so-good days

Tuesday, Week 1

Units allowed: 2 Milk, 4 Vegetable, 3 Fruit, 6 Bread, 7 Meat, 2-3 Fat
Calories allowed: 1,500

time	food eaten	calories
7:30 A.M.	8 ounces water on rising	
7:45 A.M.	4 ounces skim milk in de-caffeinated cappuccino (½ Milk)	43
	1 slice protein toast (½ Bread)	40
	1 teaspoon butter (1 Fat)	45
	1 egg, poached (1 Meat)	75
9:05 A.M.	8 ounces decaffeinated tea with lemon (Free)	
	6 ounces water and vitamins	
11:15 A.M.	1 fairly large apple (2 Fruit)	80
1:00 P.M.	8 ounces water before meal	
	1 cup strawberry yogurt (2 Milk)	170
	1 cube of cornbread (1 Bread)	70
3:30 P.M.	1 small bran muffin (1 Bread)	70
	8 ounces decaffeinated tea with lemon (Free)	
5:30 P.M.	small salad of alfalfa sprouts and shredded carrots, with rice-vinegar and soy sauce dressing (1 Vegetable)	25
	1 cube of cornbread (1 Bread)	70
7:40 P.M.	8 ounces water before meal	
	5 ounces veal in stew (5 Meat)	375
	assorted stew vegetables (2 Vegetables)	50
	4 ounces tomato juice (1 Vegetable)	25
	1 small potato in stew (1 Bread)	70
	1 slice whole-wheat (1 Bread)	70
	1 cup plain yogurt (1 Milk)	85

10:00 P.M.   ½ small banana (1 Fruit)   40
             8 ounces chamomile tea
             (Free)
11:30 P.M.   8 ounces water
             before bed   ———

                             total: 1,403
                           deposit: 97

Units eaten: 3½ Milk, 4 Vegetable, 3 Fruit, 5½ Bread,
6 Meat, 1 Fat

ANALYSIS, TUESDAY, WEEK 1

I had an all-day booking today. But I was smart enough to plan. I brought a whole bunch of reasonable, fairly low-calorie foods along. I didn't want to get stuck eating the fattening cakes they have at the studio or any of the big lunches ordered from a nearby restaurant. My filling early morning meal helped to control my appetite and lessen the temptation to grab for the wrong thing.

In my first meal of the day, I ate a slice of high-protein bread, which was recorded as a half unit rather than a full unit. This bread simply has less carbohydrates per slice and therefore about half the calories. It's a good way to stretch your Bread units. But then, I found myself almost overdoing the Bread units for most of the day. A neighbor had stopped by in the morning with a large pan of cornbread. I *love cornbread!* I took a piece with me to work and had another with my salad at 5:30 P.M. when I came home. Just before my friend showed up for dinner, I decided to make the remainder of the cornbread a present to her. So, I wrapped it up in tin foil and put it away for later. Not bad— avoiding calories and coming off as a generous soul.

It was great seeing my friend. Dinner was so complete and satisfying she didn't even realize I was cutting down. Granted, this was more extensive than your typical minimeal. But this is a *flexible* food plan. Special occasions call for slight deviations from the norm.

In truth, I ate more food today overall than I did yesterday. My Milk units went a little over the amount allowed, and the nutritional balance for the day might have suffered. Yet I stayed under the one thousand five hundred-calorie limit. In a few instances I showed good judgment and constraint. Basically, most of the food I ate was healthy.

Speaking of healthy intake, I've also been trying to wean myself off of caffeine products the last two days. My cappuccino and teas were caffeine free. I skipped colas, chocolate, and all those diet beverages, too. Caffeine has a tendency to accumulate in your intestines. It can prevent your system from absorbing the nutrients provided by other foods you eat.

Taking everything into consideration, I'd say this was another relatively successful day.

PROGRESS REPORT, END OF WEEK 1

Sunday. The first week has just flown by. My minimeal routine has become a lot more comfortable in the last few days. I believe my stomach is already shrinking. I look forward to eating something every two hours or so, but the large meals seem like an awful burden. Even big portions (offered now and then) strike me the wrong way.

At a glance my tummy appears a little flatter, and I'm building up the courage right now to weigh myself. I'd hate to let the numbers of a scale ruin the sense of momentum. So far, I've gone over 1,500 calories only once—by 26 insignificant calories. Most of the other days ended in the 1,300 to 1,400 range. Listen, I'm dumping 933 unused calories out of my savings envelope today. It makes me rather proud. Yet, I'm left with a sort of bittersweet feeling.

The exercising has combined with the food plan to totally eliminate late-afternoon or early evening naps. In general, I'm more energetic and alert. On Friday and Saturday my after-workout meal was reduced to some bouillon soup and an apple. I guess late-afternoon hunger is also disappearing. At night, I sleep soundly and so does my tummy.

Okay, it's time to hit the old scale. Hey, give me a fanfare! I've lost just about four pounds!

ANN'S OH-SO-GOOD DAYS

Friday, Week 2

Units allowed: 2 Milk, 4 Vegetable, 3 Fruit, 6 Bread, 7 Meat, 2-3 Fat
Calories allowed: 1,500

time	food eaten	calories
8:05 A.M.	8 ounces water on rising	
8:30 A.M.	¼ cantaloupe (6-inch diameter) (1 Fruit)	40
	½ cup cooked farina (1 Bread)	70
	4 ounces skim milk in decaffeinated cappuccino (½ Milk)	43
11:00 A.M.	8 ounces water and vitamins	
	½ cup tuna in water (2 Meat)	150
	2 krisp toasts (1 Bread)	70
	1 heart of palm	
	½ roast pepper	
	2 leaves romaine lettuce (1 Vegetable)	30
	6 ounces seltzer with lime (Free)	
2:05 P.M.	8 ounces chicken bouillon with 1 teaspoon miso, bean sprouts, and tofu (½ Meat)	38
	1 small orange (1 Fruit)	40
4:30 P.M.	½ cup coffee ice milk (1½ Milk)	125
6:15 P.M.	1 sesame toast (½ Bread)	35
	1 tablespoon cream cheese (1 Fat)	45
	8 ounces decaffeinated coffee, black (Free)	
8:30 P.M.	5 ounces broiled swordfish steak (5 Meat)	375
	1 small baked potato (1 Bread)	70
	1 teaspoon butter (1 Fat)	45
	steamed escarole, zucchini, carrots (3 Vegetable)	75
	6 ounces seltzer with lime (Free)	
	1 cup strawberries, fresh, no sugar (1 Fruit)	40
11:30 P.M.	8 ounces mint herbal tea (Free)	
12:30 A.M.	8 ounces water before bed	
	total:	1,291
	deposit:	209

Units eaten: 2 Milk, 4 Vegetable, 3 Fruit, 3½ Bread, 7½ Meat, 2 Fat

ANALYSIS, FRIDAY, WEEK 2

The longer the food plan goes on, the more gimmicks I look to try. Recently, I've been opening or closing most minimeals with fruit. They're tasty, and at forty calories a unit you can't find a more economic dessert. Fresh fruits are usually best, but be sure to check what's in season. Avoid the canned fruit packed in the fattening heavy syrup.

Tuna eaters should also watch out for fish that's packed in thick oil. You'll be getting a lighter, lower-calorie product when the tuna is floating in water. As a rule, I've found label reading to be a necessity. I'm astounded by all the hidden calories and unhealthy byproducts that usually go unnoticed. Don't let words like *sucrose, corn syrup, malt, dextrose, salt,* or *sugar* just slip by. I'm now scanning packages for the calories-per-serving information, too.

Today's menu came across so full and *filling*! I was surprised that my one thousand five hundred-calorie allowance wasn't completely gone by the time I met my friends for a restaurant dinner. This morning's hot farina was a heftier dish than you'd expect for only seventy calories. My eleven-o'clock tuna salad offered three kinds of vegetables for little more than the calories found in just one unit. A half cup of ice milk after recreation gave me all the satisfaction of more fattening ice cream. And my Free chicken bouillon was transformed into a sumptuous specialty by adding thirty eight calories worth of sprouts, tofu (soybean curd), and a dash of Japanese miso (fermented soybean paste).

However, a full-blown dinner should have put me way over the calorie top. Deep down I was almost tickled by the idea of spending some of my surplus calories. I didn't like just letting them go at the end of a week. But my now-calorie-conscious eating habits just took over. I did the right things almost in spite of myself.

The swordfish steak they brought me was at least eight ounces. So I automatically cut away a piece and shoved it to the side of my plate. Then I put the potato and vegetables into the same plate as the swordfish. This made the portions look bigger and therefore seem more satisfying. I drank bubbly seltzer with a twist of lime—a dead ringer for many alcoholic mixes. At the end, ordering fresh strawberries without anything on them seemed to be the easiest part of all.

Voilà! I turned a sure deficit into another sizable surplus.

PROGRESS REPORT, END OF WEEK 2

Sunday. My low-calorie instincts finally fell down on the job. On Saturday, I used up quite a few of those coveted surplus calories. It took a party atmosphere, a couple of mixed drinks, and an outrageous buffet to put me 500 calories over my daily limit. This morning I feel pretty guilty. But logically there's no reason why I should. Oh well, I'm still staring at a savings envelope with 803 never-to-be-spent calories.

Going so far over the top this once may be a good thing in the long run. Now I've got it out of my system, and next week should be the best yet. I can't believe how stuffed my stomach felt last night. My tummy has definitely shrunk, because it previously took a lot more food to bring on discomfort. Maybe I'll do a little extra pep-stepping tomorrow to make up for it.

Earlier in this week, I had a really good time cooking. I prepared some fabulous ethnic foods and got a kick out of adapting the recipes to my needs. If you're a budding chef, try your hand at converting fattening dishes into slenderizing treats. You'll be amazed by what you can do. Later on, I'll share some delicious low-cal creations of my own with you.

I'm not getting on the scale today. My period is due, and I refuse to be disappointed by a temporary water retention. I'd rather think positive; just forge ahead. After all, my calorie totals don't lie!

ANN'S OH-SO-GOOD DAYS

Sunday, Week 3

Units allowed: 2 Milk, 4 Vegetable, 3 Fruit, 6 Bread, 7 Meat, 2-3 Fat
Calories allowed: 1,500

time	food eaten	calories
8:45 A.M.	8 ounces water on rising	
9:10 A.M.	¼ cantaloupe (6-inch diameter) (1 Fruit)	40
	1 whole-wheat English muffin (1 Bread)	70
	tea with lemon (Free)	
10:50 A.M.	6 ounces water and vitamins	
	1 cup puffed-wheat cereal (1⅓ Bread)	100
	½ small banana (1 Fruit)	40
	4 ounces skim milk (½ Milk)	43

12:45 P.M.	½ small spaghetti squash (1 Vegetable)	25
	2 tablespoons tomato sauce (2 Vegetable)	50
	cup of decaffeinated coffee, black (Free)	
3:00 P.M.	1 tablespoon peanut butter (1 Meat)	75
	1 slice whole-wheat bread (1 bread)	70
	6 ounces seltzer with lemon (Free)	
5:05 P.M.	8 ounces water before meal	
	8 ounces chinese cabbage (1 Vegetable)	25
	1 tablespoon blue-cheese dressing (1 Fat and ½ Milk)	85
7:30 P.M.	½ cup each of carrots, zucchini, onions, and mushrooms (4 Vegetables)	100
	1 ounce melted muenster cheese (1 Fat)	45
	8 ounces tea with lemon (Free)	
8:30 P.M.	1 cup applesauce (2 Fruit)	80
9:45 P.M.	6 ounces ice milk, vanilla (2 Milk)	170
10:40 P.M.	8 ounces water before bed	
	total:	1,018
	deposit:	482

Units eaten: 3 Milk, 8 Vegetable, 4 Fruit, 3⅓ Bread, 1 Meat, 2 Fat

ANALYSIS, SUNDAY, WEEK 3

This was the last day of the program. Even though I had 1,107 calories on deposit, I wanted to finish off real strong. So, I decided to make today a tribute to complex carbo-hydrates. I ate a lot of veggies, fruit, and some whole-grain bread and cereal.

Contrary to popular belief, all these complex carbohydrates help in weight control. They fill you up, provide a quick source of energy, and go relatively light on the calories. Sure, I had a whopping eight units of Vegetables. But together they only add up to 200 calories. In contrast, I easily gave up quite a few Meat and Bread units that have a much higher concentration of calories. That explains an enjoyable eating day with a meager 1,018 calories as the price.

My nutrition balance for today appears to be horrendous. Actually, it's not as bad as it looks. Most of us have a tendency to consume too much protein every day. Ideally, carbohydrates should account for a higher percentage of our daily intake than protein. It doesn't hurt to tip the scales back the other way every once in a while. Of course, consistently balanced eating is best.

One more comment on the day. I know that 6 ounces of vanilla ice milk came too late at night, put me over the limit for Milk units, and chalked up too many unnecessary calories. Well, I don't care. It was my way of celebrating the end of a successful shape-up cycle. Heck, I deserved it!

PROGRESS REPORT, END OF WEEK 3

Sunday. The three-week cycle is over, but I'm going to continue keeping my diary. I like monitoring myself. It gives me a sense of personal power and self-control. Those hard-to-get-rid-of bad habits have a way of sneaking back into one's life. I want to see them coming.

Christmas is around the corner. I'd love to go through the holiday on the food plan. In fact, my first inclination was to start on another three-week cycle immediately. I found the demands got easier and easier to satisfy as time went on. But the pressures of Christmas might be more than my one thousand five hundred calories could withstand. So, I'll just fall back on the maintenance plan until the Yuletide season passes. The extra calories allowed will make a world of difference.

Those catalog photographers I was worrying about pleasing should love the results of my shape-up program. They can put away their extra-wide lenses. Dresses from last spring fit me just fine. Pants, jeans, and even bathing suits look more flattering. What does the scale say? Well, I did better than I expected. I've dropped a total of *eight pounds* for the three weeks.

CALORIE SAVING IN THE KITCHEN

By now you should sense that a truly successful food plan begins in the kitchen. Yes, you can get away with a couple of restaurant meals here and there. But, for the most part, you have to maintain a hands-on control of what you eat. This means learning some of the calorie saving preparation tricks first. Then, later, you can try coming up with enough variety to make your daily fare interesting.

I'm not saying you must be a gourmet chef to lose weight. Just the idea of it sounds a bit absurd. I simply want you to be aware of ingredients, combinations, calories, and alternatives. Go into the kitchen and the diningroom with your eyes open and your wits about you. Here's some of my helpful kitchen hints to start you thinking in the correct vein.

Tips on food selection and preparation

Get a pencil and paper. You might want to hang the following gems up over the kitchen cabinet.

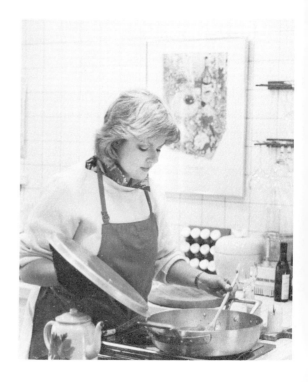

☐ Buy vegetables and fruits *fresh* whenever you can. Estimate what you'll need for the next day or two. Only buy what fits your needs and the food plan.

☐ Try to avoid buying processed foods; they often contain hidden calories.

☐ Remember, white meats—such as fish and poultry—have less calories. They also have less cholesterol.

☐ Keep to lean meats. Cut off all visible fat. Take the skin off poultry before cooking. Skim excess fat from soups by chilling them and then whisking along the surface.

☐ Try cooking with dry wines. Most of the calorie-rich alcohol evaporates in the process, yet it leaves a wonderful flavor. Sweet wines leave sugar and more calories.

☐ Wash oil-packed fish under hot water.

☐ Don't cook with oils. If you must use oil, be precise in measuring it. Oil is high in calorie content.

☐ Get into the habit of buying low-fat products—especially milk and cheeses.

☐ Don't use frozen or canned fruit that contains sugar. The same is true of fruit juices or drinks.

☐ Use vegetables in raw form whenever possible.

Soak in a solution of one part cider vinegar to sixteen parts water to remove toxins from pesticides.

☐ Make your own substitute soft drinks to replace high-calorie or high-caffeine sodas. Mix seltzer with fruit juices, such as grape and orange.

☐ Use small plates to make tiny portions look larger.

☐ Try to make acceptable foods as attractive as you can.

☐ Save for snacks the leftovers from allowable foods *only* .

Ann's lightweight, tummy-pleasing recipes

Here are some of my favorite recipes, given in conventional cookbook style. They should provide variety, help you eat more healthfully, and keep you well within the calorie range of the food plan. Several of these are obviously "company" dishes, but they're easily broken down by portion. You'll have no trouble figuring out the units consumed by an individual. Bon Appétit!

SALAD, SOUP, QUICHE, AND BREAD

Spinach salad with mushrooms and Georgie's blue-cheese dressing

½ pound fresh spinach
1 cup sliced raw mushrooms
1 cup low-fat yogurt
¼ cup blue cheese
juice of 1 lemon

Clean spinach and mushrooms and chill in refrigerator. Blend the yogurt, blue cheese, and lemon juice in a blender. Pour dressing over the combined spinach and mushrooms. *Serves 4.*

Chicken salad with broccoli

SALAD

2 whole boneless and skinless chicken breasts
1 head broccoli, flowerettes only
4 scallions
curly leaf lettuce

DRESSING

½ cup low-cal soyonnaise (available in health food stores)
1 teaspoon dried dill or 2 tblsp. fresh dill
1 teaspoon seasoned salt
fresh ground pepper to taste
paprika for garnish

Bring 2 cups water to boil in saucepan. Add chicken breasts and simmer until cooked, about 15 minutes. Let cool. Parboil broccoli for 3 minutes. Rinse under cold water. Shred or cut chicken into bite-size pieces. Cut scallions into pieces, using all but the very ends. Mix chicken, broccoli, scallions, and dressing ingredients together and chill until time to serve. Serve on a bed of curly leaf lettuce. Sprinkle with paprika for garnish. *Serves 4.*

Quick Chinese chicken soup

8 Chinese cloud ears
(or regular mushrooms, if unavailable)
2 quarts water
4 chicken bouillon cubes (low salt)
16 Chinese-snow-pea pods
1 block tofu (soybean curd), cubed
1 cup mung bean sprouts
2-4 scallions sliced

Cover cloud ears with water and soak until soft. Rinse and set aside. Bring chicken broth and water to boil. When boiling, lower heat, add remaining ingredients (including cloud ears) and simmer for 2 minutes. *Serves 4 (in bowls) or 8 (in cups).*

Curried chicken salad

SALAD

2 whole boneless and skinless chicken breasts
½ cantaloupe or available melon, cubed
½ cup unsalted sunflower seeds
½ cup currants or raisins
curly leaf lettuce

DRESSING

½ cup low-cal soyonnaise
1 tablespoon curry powder, or to taste
½ cup unsweetened coconut for garnish

Bring 2 cups water to boil in saucepan. Add chicken breasts and simmer until cooked, about 15 minutes. Let cool. Shred or cut chicken into bite-size pieces. Mix together all ingredients but coconut and chill until needed. Serve on a bed of curly leaf lettuce and garnish top with coconut. *Serves 4.*

Spinach quiche

spray-on vegetable shortening from pump dispenser (you use less so there are fewer calories)
1 package chopped frozen spinach, cooked and well drained
8 ounces low-fat cottage cheese
4 ounces plain low-fat yogurt
¼ cup plus 1 tablespoon grated parmesan cheese
4 large eggs, beaten (organic, if possible)
1 medium onion, chopped
½ teaspoon dill
¼ teaspoon nutmeg

Preheat oven to 350°. Spray a 9-inch quiche pan with shortening. Combine all ingredients, reserving 1 tablespoon parmesan cheese. Pour into quiche pan and sprinkle with reserved grated cheese. Bake for 50 minutes or until quiche puffs and knife comes out clean. *Serves 8.*

Garlic whole wheat pita bread

2-3 tablespoons garlic, minced
4 tablespoons olive oil
8 whole wheat pita

Combine garlic and oil until smooth. Split each pita open and spread a thin coating on each half. Place on foil and broil until golden brown. (You can freeze unused pita. Put a piece of foil or wax paper between each piece, then wrap.) *½ pita per serving.*

Vegetables

Stir-fried broccoli with onions

1 tablespoon peanut, safflower, or vegetable oil (cold processed)
1 tablespoon white wine
½ cup vegetable bouillon stock
2 tablespoons soy sauce
½ teaspoon unfiltered raw honey
1 teaspoon arrowroot
1 clove garlic, minced
1 teaspoon fresh ginger, minced
1 head broccoli, cut into 1-inch pieces
1 medium onion, quartered

Heat oil in a wok until a drop of water sizzles when added. Combine white wine, stock, soy sauce, honey, and arrowroot and set aside. Add garlic and ginger to heated wok. Stir fry 5 seconds. Add broccoli, raise heat, and stir fry 3 minutes. Add onion, stir fry 1 minute, then pour combined liquids into wok and stir well. Cover and cook for 3 minutes or until sauce thickens. This goes well with Marinated Chinese Chicken and brown rice. *Serves 4.*

Brown rice with carrots

1 cup brown rice
2 cups water
2 vegetable or chicken bouillon cubes
2 tablespoons water
3 medium carrots, grated
1 clove garlic, minced

Simmer rice, water, and bouillon cubes on low heat in small saucepan about 15 minutes or until water is absorbed. Add 2 tablespoons water, grated carrots, and garlic. Mix evenly into rice and simmer 5 minutes more. This goes well with broiled fish. *Serves 4.*

Baked potato skins

4 potatoes
1 tablespoon raw butter, melted
freshly ground pepper

Scrub potatoes well. Cut in half lengthwise. Using a small melon scoop, remove potato from skins, leaving about ¼ inch next to skin (save potato for other use). Brush inside of skin with melted butter, pepper to taste. Bake at 375° for about 30 minutes or until browned and crispy. *Serves 8.*

Zucchini with tomato sauce

1 small or medium zucchini per portion, scrubbed and sliced into ¼-inch rounds

Steam 5-7 minutes. Top with 2 tablespoons tomato sauce per portion.

Spaghetti squash with tomato sauce

1 1-pound spaghetti squash, cut in half, seeds removed
Microwave: Place each half in a glass dish and microwave on high setting for 6-8 minutes. Skin should pull away easily with fork.
Baked: Prick skin with fork. Place cut side down in roasting pan with 1 inch water. Bake in 350° oven for 30 minutes. Test with fork for doneness. If not cooked, turn halves over and cook, covered, 15 minutes more.

Pour tomato sauce in cavity and serve in place of spaghetti. *Serves 2.*

Green beans with tomato sauce

TOMATO SAUCE

1 16-ounce can plum tomatoes with basil
3 cloves garlic, minced
1 medium onion, chopped
¼ teaspoon crushed red pepper
1/3 cup chopped Italian (flat-leaf) parsley
3-4 leaves fresh basil, chopped,
or ¼ teaspoon dried
¼ teaspoon oregano
1 bay leaf

In a large saucepan combine all ingredients. Crush tomatoes against the side of the pan with a wooden spoon. Simmer on low heat for 1 hour. This sauce can be used for pasta, fish, chicken, or vegetables.

1 handful of green beans per portion, halved or whole

Trim ends of beans and steam for 7 to 10 minutes. Top with 2 tablespoons tomato sauce per portion.

CHICKEN, VEAL, AND FISH

Marinated Italian chicken

MARINADE

1½ cups red wine vinegar
2 teaspoons oregano
1 teaspoon basil
4 cloves garlic, minced
1 bay leaf, crushed
pepper to taste
1 3-pound chicken, skin removed, cut into 8 serving pieces
spray-on vegetable shortening (pump dispenser)

Combine all ingredients for marinade. Place chicken pieces in marinade for at least 3 hours, or, preferably, overnight. When chicken is well marinated, place pieces in baking pan that has been sprayed with shortening. Bake for 45 minutes at 400°. This is good barbecued, too. *Serves 4.*

Marinated Chinese chicken

MARINADE

½ cup rice vinegar
¼ cup soy sauce
4 cloves garlic, minced
1 tablespoon minced fresh ginger
½ teaspoon Chinese five-spice powder
1 3-pound chicken, skin removed, cut into 8 serving pieces
½ cup sesame seeds
spray-on vegetable shortening (pump dispenser)

Combine ingredients for marinade. Place chicken in marinade for 3 hours or overnight. When marinated, dip the top side of chicken pieces in sesame seeds. Then put chicken into presprayed baking pan and bake for 45 minutes at 400°. This is also good for barbecuing. *Serves 4.*

Chicken with couscous

1 pound boneless, skinless chicken breast, cubed
2 large onions, chopped
2 turnips, quartered
2 large carrots, sliced
½ teaspoon ginger
¼ teaspoon tumeric
pinch saffron
1 cup raisins
1 20-ounce can chick peas with liquid
3 small zucchini, cubed
3 tomatoes or 1 small can stewed tomatoes
5 tablespoons chopped parsley
1 pound couscous

Put chicken, onions, turnips, and carrots into a large pot. Season with ginger, tumeric, and saffron. Add water to cover. Cover and bring to a boil, then simmer 1 hour. Add raisins, chick peas, zucchini, tomatoes, and parsley. At the same time, fit a metal colander over the stew. Moisten couscous and work with fingers to eliminate lumps. Place the couscous in the colander and steam over stew for 30 minutes.

Remove couscous from colander and place in a large bowl. Break up any lumps with a wooden spoon. Return the couscous to the colander and steam over stew for 30 minutes more.

When done, take a cup of stew juice, add cayenne or chili and paprika to taste. It should be hot and spicy.

Spoon couscous onto a large serving platter. Moisten with remaining stew broth. Place stew on top of couscous and serve with the hot sauce on the side. *Serves 6.*

(If you don't want to make the couscous, this can be served with brown rice.)

Chicken breasts in mustard sauce

2 whole boneless, skinless chicken breasts
1 cup dry vermouth
2 cloves garlic, minced
2 tablespoons dried tarragon
½ cup chicken stock
½ cup low-fat yogurt
pepper to taste
1 tablespoon Dijon mustard

Cut each whole chicken breast in half to make four pieces. Bring vermouth, garlic, and 1 teaspoon tarragon to a boil in a skillet. Add chicken and lower heat to a simmer. Poach chicken about 7 minutes. Don't overcook. Set chicken aside. Add all remaining ingredients except mustard to pan and reduce sauce over medium heat, stirring constantly until consistency becomes somewhat creamy. Add mustard to sauce and return chicken to pan to reheat. This can be great served cold, too. It also goes well with green beans and wild rice. *Serves 4.*

Chicken parmigiana

2 boneless, skinless chicken breasts
3-4 tablespoons tomato sauce
4 ounces grated low-fat mozzarella cheese

In a glass baking dish (or individual serving dishes) place pounded chicken breasts in a row. Spoon homemade or sugar-free prepared tomato sauce over breasts. Top with cheese. Bake in 400° oven for 30 minutes or microwave on high setting 5-6 minutes or 1 minute per ounce of chicken. *Serves 4.*

Veal marsala with grapes

4 2-ounce veal cutlets
3 shallots, minced
¼ teaspoon tarragon
½ cup Marsala wine
1 cup seedless white grapes

Pound veal until thin. Place all ingredients but grapes in pan. Bring to boil, then simmer 3 minutes on each side. Add grapes. Cook until heated through. Serve with rice and carrots. *Serves 2.*

Veal stew

2 bay leaves
1 pound veal stew-meat, cubed
3 medium carrots, sliced in ½-inch rounds
2 medium zucchini, sliced in ½-inch rounds
3 small onions, quartered
1 ounce dried cepe mushrooms (available in specialty shops) or ¼ pound fresh regular mushrooms
2 stalks celery, sliced in ½-inch pieces
pepper to taste
4 cubes beef bouillon or 1 package onion soup mix
1½ cups water
1½ cups low-fat yogurt
1 teaspoon arrowroot

Put all ingredients into crock pot or large stew pot. Stir with spoon to blend ingredients. Cook on low heat until meat is tender, about 1 hour. Serve with brown rice or bulgur. *Serves 4.*

Baked stuffed fish fillets

STUFFING

1 pound fresh spinach (or kale), cooked
½ cup wheat germ or bran
½ cup chopped onions
¼ cup chopped water chestnuts
1/8 teaspoon nutmeg
½ cup shredded low-fat
Lorraine Swiss cheese
pepper to taste
¼ cup low-fat yogurt
¼ cup parmesan cheese
1 pound fresh fillets (4 pieces, about 4 ounces each)
paprika
juice of 1 lemon

Spray glass baking dish with spray-on vegetable shortening. Combine ingredients for stuffing. Preheat oven to 375°. Place fillets flat on a piece of wax paper. Spoon 2 table-spoons of mixture at wide end of each fillet. Roll and place seam side down in glass baking dish. Cover loosely with foil. Bake for 25 minutes. Sprinkle with lemon juice and paprika. This is good served with steamed vegetables and brown rice. *Serves 4.*

Oriental fish baked in foil

1 teaspoon minced fresh ginger
1 teaspoon minced garlic
1 tablespoon black-bean sauce (available in Chinese grocery store)
2 tablespoons soy sauce
3 tablespoons white wine
1½ pounds low-fat fish of your choice (scrod, halibut, cod, sole, flounder) or fish steaks equaling 1½ pounds
scallions (cut on diagonal) for garnish

Preheat oven to 375°. Combine spices, sauces, and wine. Put 3 tablespoons mixture on a piece of aluminum foil large enough to wrap fish up and fold edges. Slit meat of fish (on both sides if whole). Place fish on foil. Pour remainder of mixture over top of fish. Wrap ends of foil securely so nothing leaks. Bake for 25 minutes. Check for doneness by inserting fork into thicker part of fish. If flesh moves away from bone easily, then it is done. Place on platter and garnish with scallions. *Serves 6.*

CHAPTER NINE

FUN EXERCISES:

THE JOYS OF

FITNESS

Come out of hiding! Put away your trusty excuses! You don't have to be afraid of the word *exercise* around here. My kind of exercise certainly won't hurt you. It's not going to be all those painful contortions you've always hated. You see, I won't be dragged into the drudgery of calisthenics, either.

My fitness program is an important part of the time I put aside for pleasure. It's a form of recreation and relaxation. Sure, the activities help tone muscles, burn calories, improve circulation, and strengthen the heart. But there's no place for push-ups, sit-ups, jumping jacks, or squat thrusts. I don't want to begin *every* session by gritting my teeth. I'd rather start off grinning.

Everything we do will resemble *fun*, not work. We'll always open up by stretching rhythmatically to music. I call this fifteen minute routine *dance flexing*. It makes you feel great, really gets the juices flowing. And it can be done alone or with friends.

Then, on most workout days, we'll go into one of several exhilarating exercises or sports. Select the activities that appeal to you and seem to fit your physical needs. Each one recommended has a sociable or playful quality. They all get you pretty much out into the world. Still, a few activities will fit your lifestyle somewhat better than the others.

One cardinal rule to fix in your find: *Don't worry about failure!* That's not the way the program works. Everybody is encouraged to move along at their own pace. There aren't any cutoff points for success; no all-seeing coaches to grade your progress from the sidelines. Goals in these activities are essentially personal and extremely *flexible*.

I will, however, suggest a loose, wide range of performance you can aim at. But that's only to provide an informal structure for your efforts. We all require a general framework and some direction to get beneficial results. Ultimately, your abilities, ambition, and enjoyment should be your basic guide to how much exercising is enough.

Another key to the program is *patience*. Please, try to set reachable goals from the beginning. Don't make yourself strain too much at first. If you get some pleasant days under your belt, you'll be more anxious to continue. It's human nature.

After all, it could take weeks, even months, to get to the level of proficiency you may desire. Rushing the process is plain silly. It's the practice and exercise along the way that ease you into shape. So just try to get into a comfortable groove. Have a good time every second you play.

MAKING THE GAME PLAN

Up to now, you've gotten a vague overview of the kind of exercising ahead. Hopefully it has stirred up a little enthusiasm. But you won't fully appreciate the program until we develop a clear game plan. We'll lay out a sane workout schedule to take you smoothly from a sedentary existence to an active lifestyle. You'll also get a rundown of the sports I've thrived on in the past. Later, I'll help you to prepare completely for each activity.

Of course, the first step in any fitness scheme is to check in with your doctor. Let him examine the condition of your heart and other vital organs. Discuss your strengths and weaknesses. Get feedback on the activities you've chosen and the particulars of the schedule. I can only give general suggestions that suit the majority of women reading this book. Your doctor has the information necessary to tailor the game plan explicitly to you.

Usually the doctor's changes are quite minor. I believe in an effective, but fairly prudent approach. At first, the dance flexing is the bulk of the program. It's a mild introduction to exercising that helps get your spine and muscles ready for the more demanding sports to come.

The initial week of the shape-up calls for doing the dance flexing on *five consecutive days*. I prefer beginning on Monday and running through to Friday. As I've mentioned previously, each stretching session takes about fifteen minutes. These aren't the kind of exercises that produce soreness. Just the opposite is true. They keep you limber enough to ease aches from other activities.

Your sports exercising is relatively minimal the first week. I suggest only *three half-hour periods* done *on alternating days*. Once again, I like starting on Monday then leapfrogging to Wednesday and Friday. Your body has a tendency to get charley horses at this stage. Alternating days will give your body a chance to recoup. Naturally, the recreation portion of your workout always comes after the dance flexing.

In the weeks that follow, everything is slowly increased. On my progressive schedule, the *second week adds a Saturday session to both* the warm-ups and the sports curriculum. That puts your back-to-back days near the end of the week and still gives you Sunday as a breather. By the time the *third week* rolls around you should be up to *seven days a week of flexing and six days of sports*. The day off from sports is usually dictated by necessity. We're all busy, busy, busy!

However, there have been times—months at a stretch—when I've done a full workout every single day. It's no big deal! Once you get going, forty-five minutes of exercise per day seems trivial. You'll actually be looking to extend an activity here and there. I always run way over on weekend bike rides.

This brings us to the sports you have to choose from. They fall into *two groups* for our purposes. *Group One* is made up of the activities I've found to be both highly effective and very convenient. These are also the easier skills to pick up. Many women tend to pursue only sports listed in this "mainstay" group.

Group Two consists of more competitive or adventurous sports. Most of these require some rudimentary instruction and a bit more practice time. I've spent months at a time totally hooked on various Group Two selections. Often the better you get at these sports the more you want to do them.

group one	group two
bicycling	tennis
pep-step walking	dancing
jumping rope	cross-country skiing
swimming	racquetball
	snorkeling

I recommend doing only one sport from Group One during the shorter first week. This will give you the time to become comfortable with the activity and make some real progress. In the second week you should add a sport from either Group One or Group Two. Try to split the four sports sessions evenly between them. For the third week you have the option to drop an activity and replace it with a new one or simply hold pat.

Don't be surprised if a certain activity seems to be on the agenda week after week. There's usually one sport that becomes a focal point for your efforts. It's the thing you do instinctively. You get a pleasant, secure sensation every time. Besides, we all want one ongoing project that allows us to make continual improvements.

LET'S GET PHYSICAL

We'll begin with the dance flexing. I'll take you step-by-step through a typical fifteen-minute warm-up. Then it's on to Group One activities. One at a time, I'll break them down into clothes and equipment necessary, a practical workout routine, and other important considerations. Since these are the mainstay sports, they deserve the extra attention. Afterward, you'll get a *brief* comment about how to get involved in each of the Group Two offerings. Remember, most of these do require some tutoring by a knowledgeable expert.

Dance flexing

Decked out in my leotard and tights (your clothes gotta stretch with ya), I begin limbering up to the hot sounds of "Private Eyes."

The whole side one of the Hall and Oates album has just the right tempo to go with the movements I have to do. You, of course, can listen to whatever turns you on. Just be sure the music flows for the full fifteen minutes.

For starters, I rhythmically click off my *neck looseners* in time to the music. My head turns all the way to the right for a beat, pauses, then comes back to a straight ahead position. Next, I turn my head to the far left and once again click it back to the face-forward pose. This sequence is repeated five times.

The other part of the neck looseners sends my head on a different route. I tilt my head back as far as it can go, hold it for a beat, and then drop it all the way forward until my chin touches my chest. Repeating this ten times removes any stiffness or tension still in your neck.

Now, I wind up the head movements with a few *head rolls*. I just let my head go down to my chest with the music, ease over toward my right shoulder, sway back and around to the left shoulder before swooping down again to my chest. Ah, let it roll that way one more time. Then reverse directions for two revolutions. You whirl away the kinks, and tighten double chins too.

The suggestive quality of the song "Private Eyes" matches up beautifully with the *shoulder rolls*. I can feel their passionate stare (let your imagination soar) as I go into my vamping gestures. I roll my right shoulder backward in a circular motion ten times. Then I shift the shoulder into a forward gear for another ten. My left shoulder goes through the same thing. No wonder why those sirens of the silver screen were in such good shape.

On to *side bends* that tone the stomach and flatten those "love handles." I put the right hand to my waist. The left arm stretches up and over to the right as I bend in that direction. You should feel the tug in your left side, especially when you give a little added pump to the music. Don't force the issue or strain too hard. Straighten up. Do this six more times before reversing to the other side for seven side bends.

Hall and Oates now sing "Mano A Mano." I imagine that a rope is dangling just above my head. Both arms raise up and, without returning to my sides, take turns reaching high for the rope. After a while, it seems as if I'm *rope climbing* at an even hand-over-hand clip. I continue for twenty reaches in all. My upper back muscles are toned with every move I make.

Leg leans are probably the most important part of your warm-up. I lift my right leg up and let the bottom portion rest on a waist-high stool. Gracefully I bend a few inches forward from the middle. This position is held for ten long beats (about 20 seconds) before switching legs. My whole hamstring is being stretched. Hamstring pulls are bad injuries that can occur during pep-stepping, tennis, or even jumping rope.

The closing moments of dance flexing are spent doing *bend overs*. I keep my legs as straight as possible. Then, bending over, I dangle my arms down toward the floor. Twenty seconds of this tugs at the ligaments of my legs and stretches out my lower back muscles. Back in a standing position, I relax by swaying to the music. Then, it's time to bend over once more.

All in all, I'm ready to boogie into whatever activity follows.

Group one sports

Here are the mainstays in my personal order of preference.

BICYCLING

Ah, here's my favorite exercise. It keeps me off of ovenlike buses or crowded trains during the summer. The rest of the year it simply gets me into the world. Bicycling also does a great job of firming up ample thighs and a deluxe derrière. After a layoff I can get back into the flow almost immediately.

The first thing you have to take care of is picking the bike that's right for your body. Frames come in nineteen-inch to twenty-six-inch sizes. Don't get a bike that's too tall for you—a certain degree of control is bound to be lost. Men's bikes tend to have sturdier frames. If you buy a bike with a horizontal bar (for men), make sure you can straddle the bike in flat shoes. There should be an inch clearance between you and the bar. Women who want to ride in skirts can consider the mixte frame, which is a compromise between the men's and women's models. Here the horizontal bar is angled a bit, but isn't the V found in women's bikes.

The seat height must also suit your body. Try sitting on the seat with the balls of your feet on the pedals. Your legs should be practically straight, but not totally extended. When your legs are fully extended, an injury to the knee can develop. By contrast, a seat that's too low will prevent you from extending far enough to achieve optimum leg strength.

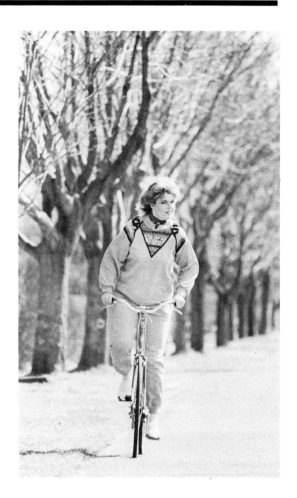

Merely loosen the nut below the seat to raise or lower it. Handlebars should also be adjusted so that your elbows are slightly bent while your hands are in place on the grips.

The idea of the bicycling exercise is to keep an even, steady rhythm for fifteen minutes at a time. After the first ride find a pleasant place to relax for five minutes. Then turn around and pedal steadily back for another fifteen minutes. Don't try to sprint for the full distance. Fifty to seventy revolutions per minute is perfect for beginners. You can gradually increase your rate of speed as your leg strength builds. Use the lower gears to make pedaling easier.

Warm up to your ride by starting slowly and easing into your own pace. Be sure to do some cooling down exercises after the ride is over. Stretch your legs in particular so that they don't tighten up. Concentrate on those hamstrings (leg leans) and calves (bend overs and massaging).

For bicycling, shorts, culottes, or pedal pushers are fine to wear during warmer weather. In chillier months try pants that gather at the ankles. This will prevent any chain entanglements. Wear bright or light colors that are readily visible to drivers. On top, wear a few lightweight layers so that you can strip down as your body heat rises.

When it's cold or snowy I hop on my old stationary bicycle. It's not as scenic as a mobile bike, but it surely fills the winter gaps. You can time yourself and count rpm's too.

PEP-STEP WALKING

I've found that my legs can take me almost anywhere a bike can—and then some. Take away my bicycle and I'll just go pep-stepping around town. In fact, pep-stepping allows me to see the passing parade a little more carefully. I get to soak up every detail of what's around me. Pep-stepping is a quick-paced walk that maintains a steady pace and develops a peppy rhythm.

Notice, I say pep-stepping instead of jogging or running. Why? Well, every single time a runner's foot hits the ground, her frame receives a shock of up to triple her body weight. A large woman could sustain serious injuries to her knees by running on the wrong surface. Yet walking briskly is just as beneficial to the heart and body as jogging. And you're not risking your knees.

The gear you wear for pep-step walking is the same as what you would find on a serious runner. I recommend a pair of running shorts and a T-shirt. Don't just borrow these from your boyfriend. Make sure the shorts fit in the crotch area and ease over any thigh bulges. They should also cover your fanny. Move around in them while you're trying them on. Be certain nothing is rubbing against flesh.

I personally prefer shorts with side slits. They're more comfortable, and further adjustments can be made on your own. Stay away from really tight waistbands that dig in, while making your tummy look bigger. Tennis sneakers or running shoes are a must for your feet. Sweat socks or peds should help to ward off blisters. Women with long hair will need a headband to keep strands out of their eyes.

The half hour of pep-stepping is broken up just like the bicycling. You walk at a crisp, smooth pace for fifteen minutes straight. Don't

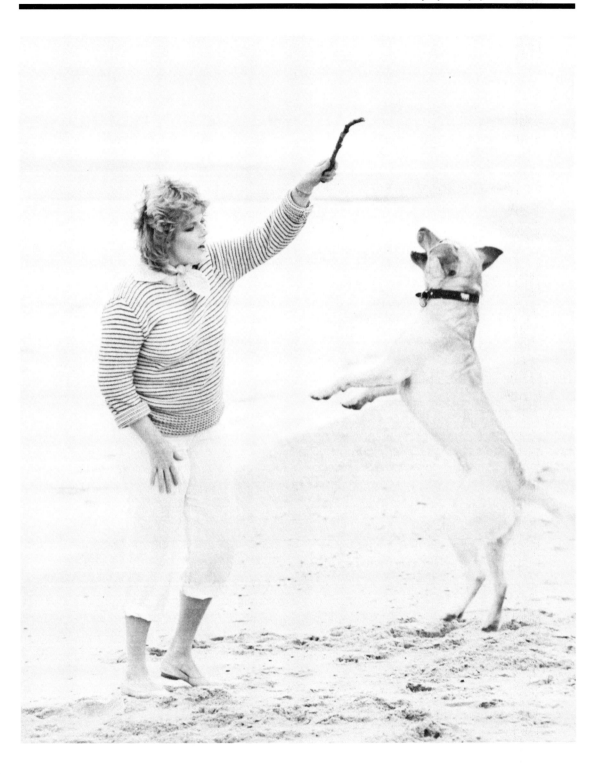

spring too much or lift your feet too high. Get into a groove, breathe in a regular cadence, and hold your arms in the same position utilized by joggers. Forget about window-shopping, ladies!

Your pep-stepping should take you to a park, pond, or maybe a beach. When you get there rest for a few minutes. Look up at the sky and take long, easy breaths. After this refreshing pause it's back on the trail. You should alter your fifteen-minute return route slightly. Always try something new.

As time goes on, either pick up your pace a drop or add a couple minutes to the round-trip walk. By your second or third shape-up cycle you should be doing as much as a half hour each way. I'm amazed by the effect pep-stepping has on my legs, thighs, fanny, and midsection. It does a lot for circulation too.

JUMPING ROPE

Little girls love it. Why shouldn't you? Actually, the image of tiny tikes skipping merrily over a rope has been outmuscled in recent years by brawny boxers rope dancing themselves into shape. Most athletes now recognize the cardiovascular, timing, wind, circulation, and calorie-burning advantages to jumping rope. It's a toy that has grown up into a fabulous form of exercise.

I was reintroduced to jumping rope during a very busy period last year. It helped make up for all the dance classes I was forced to miss while on the road. What could be more portable or convenient than a thin rope that works just as well indoors as it does in the park? I was able to carry the rope in my bag and work out between shootings or appearances.

However, not just *any* cute little jump rope will do. I think you should invest in a professional type of rope. Everlast makes a great one with a leather rope and ball bearings in the handles. Both the leather and ball bearings make it swing easier and smoother.

It's also important to get the correct length for you. The rope should be twice the distance from your armpit to the floor. Remember, the middle of the rope is what strikes the floor during a complete revolution. For the sake of measuring, double up the rope and let it dangle from just under your shoulder.

Some women protest that they're too large to jump rope. Nothing could be further from the truth. We're not talking about high leaps into the air. All you need is a few inches of clearance to allow the rope to pass beneath your feet. It's a subtle, understated kind of bobbing that comes from bouncing on the balls of your feet. Never jump flat-footed!

Spend the first workout session just getting used to controlling the rope. Practice maintaining a roll and keeping a steady cadence. Go slowly; let your feet feel the rhythm. Music is a wonderful aid in the beginning. It emphasizes the underlying beat and timing.

For the rest of the week try to work up to two minutes of nonstop jumping. Aim for four nonstop minutes by the end of the second week. Use your full session to strive for your goal. You would be surprised how those one- and two-minute attempts add up in the course of a half hour. By the third week set your sights on an easy-going, nonstop roll of five minutes. Don't be disappointed if you fall short. Believe me, five minutes without a breather is the big time.

The long, long-range goal of any serious rope jumper is to skip evenly through fifteen uninterrupted minutes. I'm still only about halfway there. But the path to success is relatively smooth because I dress defensively. I wear a well-supported bra to take the strain of my jiggling breasts. And I cushion the pounding by wearing sneakers or rubber-soled shoes.

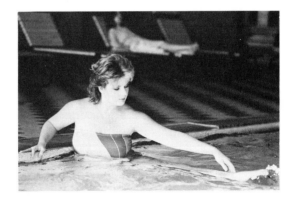

SWIMMING

Moving through the water is the best overall body toner. It's one of the few exercises that work equally on both sides of your physique. Swimming is especially good for those of us who are slightly older or really out of shape. You get a chance to work out, increase flexibility, improve balance (on land too), and strengthen your lungs. What's more, all this is accomplished without putting stress on your joints or spine.

The ideal approach to water exercising for women is *aerobic training* or distance swimming. You begin by merely swimming as far as you can before running out of gas. Please, no wild thrashing or bursts of speed. Simply cruise along with an even kick, regular breathing pattern, and relaxed stroke. Your goal is to build up to a steady fifteen minutes of nonstop swimming.

It takes a minimum of fifteen minutes to create an aerobic effect. Your heart will be strengthened considerably, and circulation is drastically improved. Don't worry about pooping out immediately or sinking to the bottom. Women are more buoyant than men for one thing. In addition, your heart pumps ten percent to twenty percent more blood with each contraction while you're in the water. So you can physically work longer and harder than you could on land.

Warm-ups are a must for swimmers. Besides the dance flexing, I advise a few more presplash maneuvers. Do some bend overs and knee bends at poolside. Maybe throw in a leg lean or two. Once you're in the water, do a very slow lap to tune up your limbs and loosen your ankles. Tense muscles tire much too quickly.

After your swimming workout take the time to cool down. A gliding lap of sidestroking is perfect. Then, oxygenate your system by totally exhaling deep breaths underwater. Repeating this several times eliminates the carbon dioxide buildup. Finally, walk around the shallow end of the pool to regain your land legs. Otherwise, you could be a little wobbly when you leave the water.

Swimming is not as inconvenient as you may think. Your local YWCA is usually close to home, relatively inexpensive, and prepared to meet your needs. Most Ys have the longer Olympic-sized pools (seventy-five feet by thirty feet), are divided into swimming lanes, and remain kiddy free for at least a few hours a day. The lifeguards and instructors available are often enthusiastic and completely willing to help you.

Please, don't back out of the swimming because you're uptight about being seen in a bathing suit. Give yourself a real chance.

Throw away those great big cover-up suits. Wear a sharp-looking suit made of spandex. It's a fabric that holds you in and masks a lot of figure faults.

Women with box shapes should try crisscrosses at the waist, high leg holes, and perhaps a sarong suit. Barrels might try suits with blouson tops and high-cut maillot-type bottoms (to show off those legs). Pear shapes and figure 8s must avoid bikinis, but can also go for maillots with the high cut. Bustier women definitely look better with underwiring for extra support.

Group two sports

I don't want to step on the toes of your prospective instructors. But I do have some quickie advice concerning the competitive or adventure sports.

TENNIS

For the purposes of exercising, approach tennis with an eye toward good ground strokes. Work at getting the kind of level swing and follow-through necessary for consistency. The idea is to have long steady volleys that keep you hopping around the court. Sure, a strong serve and devastating overhead win points. But they don't give you much of a chance to burn up calories.

In the beginning, find somebody patient enough to just volley with you. Don't even bother with playing games or keeping score. If you can spend twenty minutes a session hitting and moving for the ball, then you're doing great. Practicing your stroke against a wall is also fine for your body and game.

DANCING

There are a variety of dance classes to choose from. Again, check your neighborhood YWCA or local Yellow Pages. Large women can be graceful, rhythmic, coordinated, and quite aesthetically appealing. If I can do well in several forms of dance, so can you. Just select the type of dancing that fires your imagination and spirit.

Aerobic dancing is a good, fast-paced routine that builds cardiovascular strength, endurance, and flexibility, and firms flab. It's choreographed to include stretching, twisting, bending, *et cetera. Jazz dancing* is also an up-tempo dance form. You'll find it great for toning stomach, legs, and buttocks. I've gotten an extra kick out of *tap dancing.* A half hour of clicking away burns calories, tones legs and makes you want to buy a top hat.

CROSS-COUNTRY SKIING

Here's another one of those exercises that tone both sides of the body equally. Don't be intimidated by the narrow skis. Most women—large and not so large—find cross-country skiing extremely easy to learn. The key is to relax and get into the gliding-and-poling rhythm.

Usually you go skiing for a couple of hours at a time. I suggest keeping to rather level terrain and trying to maintain a steady pace. Balance while skiing is achieved primarily by equal and opposite motions—leg extensions and arm extensions, fore and aft, diagonally together. Work at doing a good "diagonal stride" for ten minutes at a time. Stop in between for short rests. The best clothing is knickers, a few layers of clothing on top (cotton turtleneck, flannel shirt, light sweater), flexible leather ski gloves, and a knit hat.

RACQUETBALL

This is one of the fastest-growing sports in the United States. Four-wall racquetball is played in sort of a wooden cube. It's a much faster, more intricate game than the one-wall variety. Yet, the single-wall game usually offers volleys, more exercising, and an easier adjustment for the novice.

I suggest you try both. Don't confuse the swing in racquetball with a tennis forehand or backhand. Here you're looking to use more wrist and less arm. But I'll leave that to your instructor. Just try for the long volleys again and leave your ego in the locker room. It's wonderful for your legs, waist, arms, and love handles.

SNORKELING

For those of you lucky enough to be near a beach or a clear body of water, this is a must! Besides toning your arms, legs, and midsection, you'll be discovering an awesome new world. Equipment is fairly reasonable and quite important. Don't cheap out on the fins and mask. A good pair of fins can make a huge difference in your level of enjoyment.

You probably won't need more than a single hour lesson. Afterward, try to snorkel with a friend or group. Stay moving and exploring for ten to twenty minutes at a time. Avoid zooming around aimlessly. Set routes or patterns for yourself and cover them at a smooth pace. You'll *love* it!

TAKING CARE OF YOUR BIRTHDAY SUIT

When the workout is over, a whole new shape-up begins. So far, you've concentrated on fat, muscle, vital organs, and blood circulation. It's wonderful for your insides. But now it's time to take care of your outside. Let's fix up the skin you were born in.

A not-too-hot shower follows every sports activity. (A really hot shower tends to dry out the skin.) The shower will prevent the rash called intertrigo. It comes from overactive sweat glands. Large women have been known to get intertrigo from chafing as well. Watch for it between the thighs or under your breasts.

The best way to deal with intertrigo is to clean your body with a mild soap. I like to use a minty castile soap, which is very refreshing. Be sure to dry yourself completely. Then, with a talc, powder the areas that may get rubbed. *Do not* under any circumstances substitute cornstarch for the talc. It acts as a breeding ground for bacteria and often worsens the rash.

While you're still showering, look to slough off any dead skin cells on your body. Use a loofah just about everywhere. It'll give you a rosy, lustrous glow. And, oh, how smooth you'll feel!

Callouses on your feet can be minimized with BUF-PUF. More serious buildups can be treated with a pedicure. The skin on your soles and palms is about ten times thicker than anywhere else on your body. As a result, you're safe to use a little more aggressive therapy on those spots. I've rubbed away problems with lava stones and pumices without causing any harm.

The best way to conclude a fitness program is to cream up with a light perfume-free lotion. Your skin becomes silky smooth to the touch. Then, cuddle up with someone who will appreciate your firmer body and the skin covering it. You'll feel supremely confident and as lithe as a cat.

All the passion, contact, and beautiful moments that follow are simply more of the "joys of fitness."

POSTURE AND PERK

The final phase of our shape-up program works toward healthy, attractive posture. Oh, how every fuller-figure woman needs this. It seems we've always had trouble finding the correct way to move or hold our bountiful bodies. Part of the problem has been our own self-consciousness. But plenty of people over the years have confused us with wrong directions.

Even as an oversized kid, I remember gym teachers barking orders at me. Stand up straight . . . head up . . . shoulders back . . . chest out . . . stomach in . . . fanny down! We were told that this is *perfect* posture. It was more like being drafted. Yet, many of the heavy girls I knew got right into line. Quite a few of them are still marching around as adults.

Unfortunately, the old "military stance" is far from ideal. You come across incredibly stiff, static, and awkward. What's worse, underneath the mechanical surface, stress-related ailments are flaring up from head to toe. An upturned chin compresses the neck, leading to a locked jaw or severe headaches. The forced-out chest overextends your rib cage, which can cause swayback. Sucking in your tummy stops the free flow of oxygen. Squeezing down your buttocks puts pressure on the spine. Even your legs get strained from forcing the knees back for so long.

For what it's worth, I was too uptight about thrusting out my blossoming breasts or holding in my paunch to obey the gym teachers. But the alternative I came up with was just as bad. I tried to *shrink into my own*

165

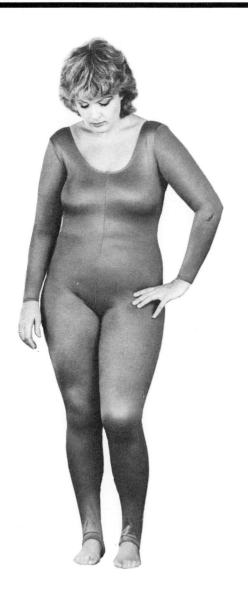

body. Sounds crazy? Well, millions of large-sized gals attempt it all the time.

You know what I mean. First, you slouch your shoulders over to appear more compact. Of course, that only makes you look squat by cutting down your height and squishing out the midsection. Hunched shoulders also pull your neck muscles, head, or both forward, creating stress in the upper back.

Next, you wind up pulling in your chest to supposedly hide the upper torso's heft. Fat chance of that fooling anybody! Your back simply gets arched, while the fanny is pushed way out. Then, you jut your hip out to draw attention away from fat legs or a broad back. The result is a distorted figure that's bent into a zigzag pattern. Any vertically streamline features become more horizontal and uneven. Again, you're making the whole body seem even heavier, strained.

I guess you're starting to see exactly why I take faulty posture so seriously. The last thing any of us wants is an inflexible, aching body crammed with trumped-up eyesores. But the remedy demands a lot of changes. You have to bring a natural quality to everything you do. Your way of walking, standing, sitting, and even reclining must be reevaluated.

We'll begin by introducing you to the theory behind proper posture. What makes it work and why? A little bit of insight here can go a long way toward success. After the theory, you'll get a point-by-point breakdown of the *truly* correct approach to the body positions mentioned previously. As a conclusion, I'll demonstrate some marvelous routines for overcoming the effects of poor posture. These were provided by exercise therapist Gail Pudaloff, director of KINETICS in New York.

Aligning your body

The key to holding your body correctly is to clearly visualize what you're aiming at. You have to sort of zoom in on a role model. Well, who can we turn to for a shining example? There is not much of a choice. Let's be honest, there aren't too many qualified candidates around.

I had to reach way back to Halloween for my posture-perfect heroine. Her name is Ms. Bones. She's a dangling skeleton who displays all the right physical attributes. Ms. Bones is quite upright, naturally loose, and her body parts hang downward in the best possible fashion.

Think of the bones of the skeleton as "building blocks" for proper posture. The blocks are all fixed into place, but they're connected by resilient pieces of elastic. This gives the dangling body flexibility and the strength to snap back. Our Ms. Bones always appears limber without flying off in every direction. She would never stiffly force her rib cage forward or poke out a misguided hip.

I'd say everything about the skeleton seems balanced. Her parts all fall along a well-centered vertical plane. That "centered" vertical plane is her *plumb line*. It's as if a weight were tied to the bottom of a string. The weight pulls the string taut, long, and absolutely straight.

When your body stacks up along its own plumb line, you're considered to be beautifully *aligned*. You should be able to draw a line down from the center of your left ear. That line would run through the middle of your shoulder to the hip. From the hip it would plunge beyond the outer center of your knee to the crease just in front of the ankle joint. This is the point where you balance the whole weight of your body.

Any detours or deviations en route mean you're out of alignment. Try to go back and get it right. Here's some help.

Taking a proper stance

Recheck your way of standing by copying my example. Don't worry about how perfect *my* posture happens to be. After all, I've thoroughly studied my friend Ms. Bones. I'm going to internally mimic her stance as closely as possible so that *every* one of my building blocks will match up to the skeleton.

As you can see from the photos, my impersonation is right on the money. Notice the vertical feeling throughout my body. It starts with my head lifted high above squared-off shoulders. The neck is lengthened and continues the vertical line downward. Yet, my chin remains parallel to the ground with a very relaxed jaw.

Like Ms. Bones, my breastbone (sternum) is *slightly* up and forward. It's supposed to be just in front of your plumb line. I also make sure that my navel lines up right above my pubic bone. This indicates that my stomach muscles are in position to help support the spine. Take a good look at your pelvic joints. If they're pointed straight ahead like the headlights of a car, you're doing fine.

My legs complete the proper standing posture by hanging long and reasonably

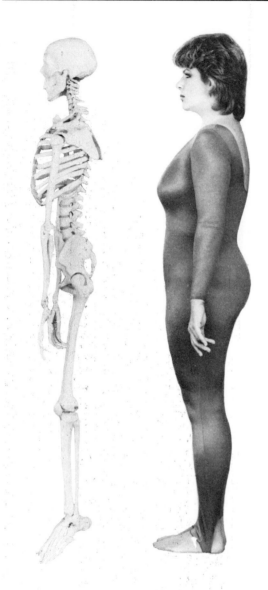

loose. Let your knees ease a bit forward so they stay unlocked. Naturally, my weight is shared by both legs evenly. You should get the feeling that a quick movement in any direction would be comfortable. Hey, I can even bob up and down like a dangling skeleton without losing my balance.

Walking like a dream

Once you're actually walking, the focal point of good posture shifts immediately to your feet. Don't get me wrong. Your body still has to remain upright, well-aligned, and balanced. But the way you use your feet can be the ultimate difference between walking like a dream or stumbling around in pain.

You can begin by thinking *nimble*. Avoid stomping your feet when you walk. Too heavy an impact will send a sharp, painful message up from your heel. That message often travels through your leg to the lower back. Some women have even stomped themselves into a succession of headaches.

The idea is to carefully plant your foot and then smoothly follow through. You must use all the muscles and ligaments in your feet. This will allow you to distribute the shock evenly. A total foot implant also keeps your feet more supple, pliant, and resilient.

I've broken a *perfect step* down into three strategic motions. Now you have to make an effort to walk by these numbers:

1   Plant your foot a half inch forward of the back of its heel.
2   Roll steadily through the center of your foot to the ball of your foot.
3   Push solidly off the toes.

Sitting pretty

Is there a real difference to the way people sit? Ask a woman who has been sitting at her desk all day. The expression on her face will be answer enough. A look of pain or discomfort means she's probably a *slumper*. If she smiles and shrugs, then the lady most likely sits comfortably tall.

Slumping into yourself is a prime example of poor sitting posture. It makes you look heavier and aggravates several areas of your body. You usually feel it in your back muscles, hip joints, and spinal column. Your head is sort of leaning forward on a slant toward the chest. This also compresses the chest, which stops your "breathing muscle" (diaphragm) from functioning efficiently.

The only way to be sitting pretty and healthy is to prop yourself up. Sit tall! Bring your torso vertical to your "sitz" (sitting) bones. You can find these by rocking back and forth in the seat; the two sharp bones sticking down are the ones.

Try to keep a minimal curve to your back. The body should resemble half of an H (ㄣ). As usual, your chin is parallel to the floor, the chest is elevated slightly, and your shoulders hang naturally. Separate your knees the width of your pelvic bone; keep feet flat on the floor. Your body must always be balanced while sitting.

Reclining in style

Did you ever wake up in the morning with a terrible pain in your lower back? Just about all of us have at one time or another. The problem is we don't sleep, rest, or recline in the proper style. There's a lot more to lying down comfortably than simply plopping onto the bed.

For starters, never sleep on your stomach. It creates too much of a curvature of your lower spine. Sleeping on your side is usually best. Resting on your back isn't too bad either.

Keep your head in line with the shoulders. Bend the knees slightly and put a pillow under your thighs. The pillow helps to get the body aligned, which takes a lot of pressure off the lower back. Use a flat pillow for your head or none at all.

You'll find yourself resting more soundly and rising with a pain-free, elongated spine.

POSTURE EXERCISES

By now you should be locked into the look and feel of proper posture. However, a lifetime of poor posture habits won't just disappear overnight. You're going to be experiencing tension, stiffness, or even pain for a while at least. So, it's time to turn to some of those therapeutic exercises I promised you earlier.

Gail Pudaloff's exercises will improve flexibility, strengthen key muscles, and help you relax. Of course, certain routines do more for specific areas of your body. Try them all or choose the ones that fit your problems. I'll demonstrate each exercise to make them easier to follow. They're the next best thing to actually being at the KINETICS body studio.

Standing cat stretch

This exercise unhinges a stiff or stuck spine. It makes your back and spine more flexible and supple.

Start off standing with your feet twelve to eighteen inches apart. Then bend forward with your spine as straight as mine. I rest my hands against bent knees. Notice how this puts me in a catlike position.

The actual exercise is done while inhaling and exhaling. I inhale slowly and begin to curl my spine under. At the same time my abdominal muscles contract into my spine. Exhaling, I continue to roll my torso upward. My hands slide up the thighs as I go. This returns me to the cat stance.

Remember to inhale as you roll up and exhale as you uncurl your spine. Repeat the exercise five to eight times. It can be done whenever you feel the need to unhinge your spine.

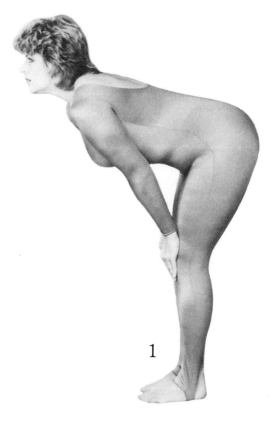

1

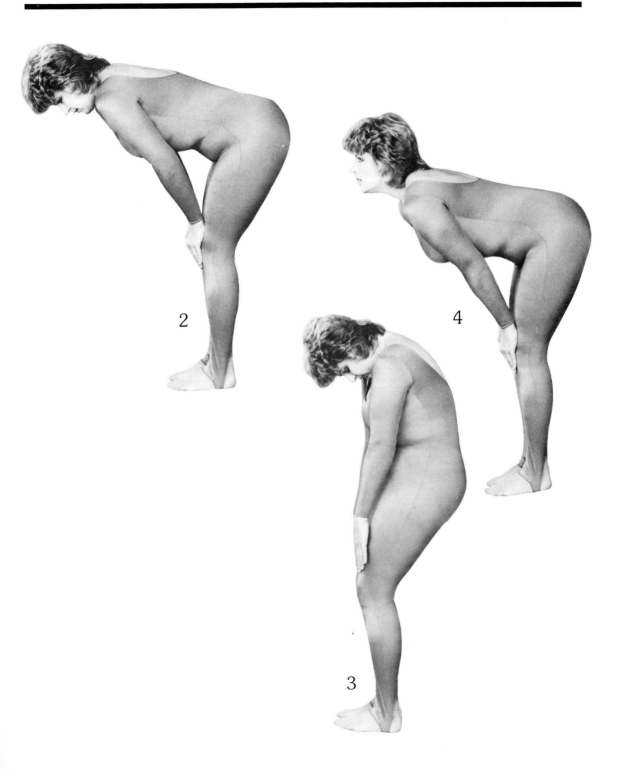

2

3

4

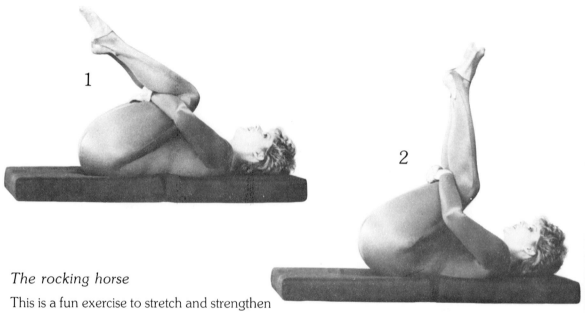

The rocking horse

This is a fun exercise to stretch and strengthen your spine. It also stimulates back muscles at the same time.

Lie on a cushioned surface and hug your knees to your chest. Check my position in the photo. Now I'm beginning to roll back to my shoulders; then forward and up to my tailbone. "Rock" in a rhythm that's steady and easy.

Complete about a dozen or so of these rocking-horse motions each time.

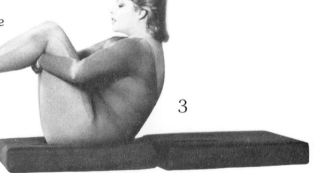

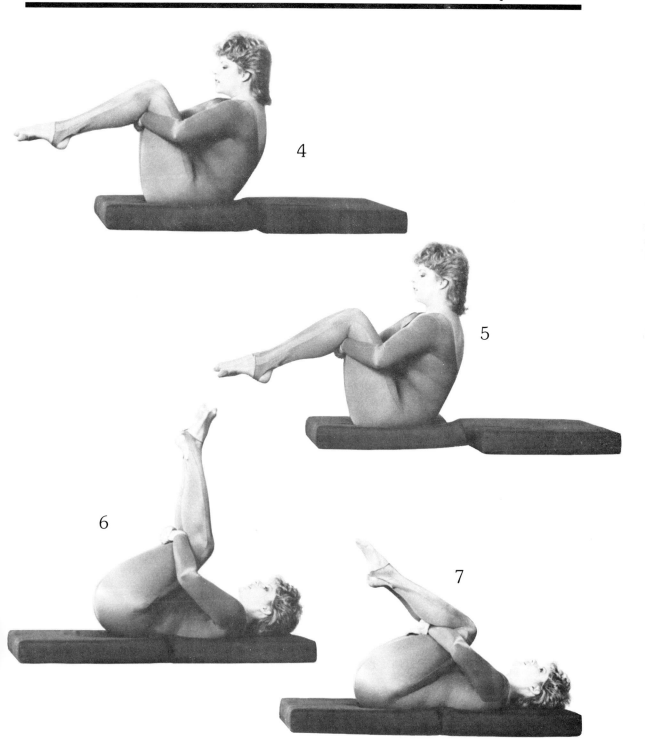

Towel behind the back

A simple, passive exercise, this stretches the chest and relieves tightness in your shoulder joints.

This exercise can be done standing or sitting. First I grasp a towel overhead in my left hand. Bending my elbow, I let the towel hang down my back. Next, I bend my right arm back and grab hold of the dangling towel. I hold this position for ten seconds breathing comfortably.

Slowly my hands "walk" toward each other on the towel. They get as close as possible before starting to move the towel up and down. It should look like I'm "buffing" my back. Repeat the process five to ten times or until your shoulders begin to unhinge.

Do it all over again with the arms reversed.

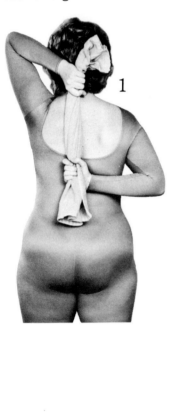
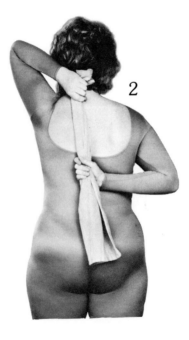
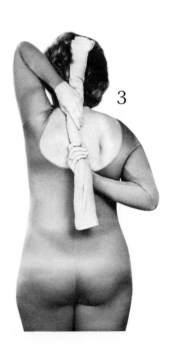

Hip and lower-back relievers

An exercise to stretch and relax the whole hip and lower-back area, it is also a great way to get relief from lower-back discomfort caused by poor posture.

I lie on my back with knees bent in toward the chest. My arms are folded under my head, palms face up. Here I do three "pelvic tilts" in a row. A pelvic tilt begins by gently inhaling as I roll my pelvis forward. This arches my back slightly off the floor. Then, exhaling I roll my back into the floor.

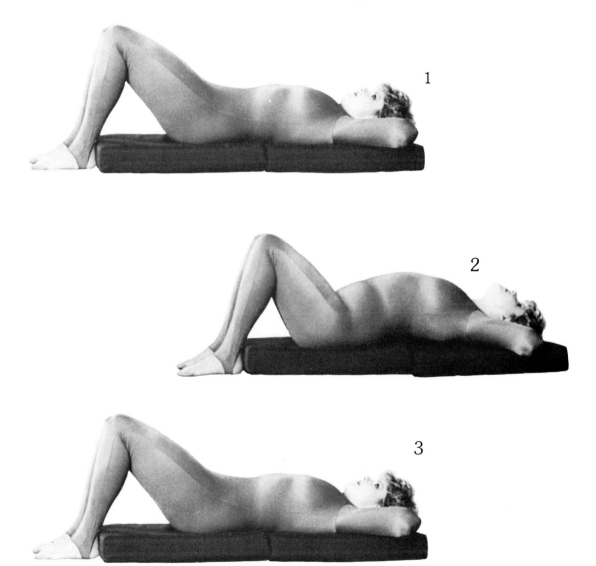

After the pelvic tilts, I elevate my knees into my chest, arms outstretched at shoulder level. I inhale and exhale three times. On the third exhale, I press my palms firmly into the floor (for stability) and rotate my knees to the right. At the same time I'm turning my head to the left.

Afterward, I rest and breathe deeply. I try to feel my back "letting go." Then I inhale and exhale, contracting the abdominals, as I lift my knees back to the center.

Do the whole thing over again working to your left. Complete five to eight sets slowly with deep breathing throughout.

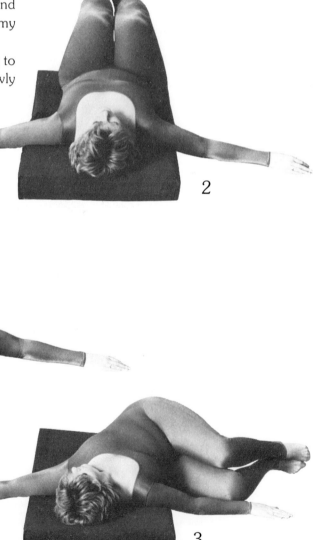

2

1

3

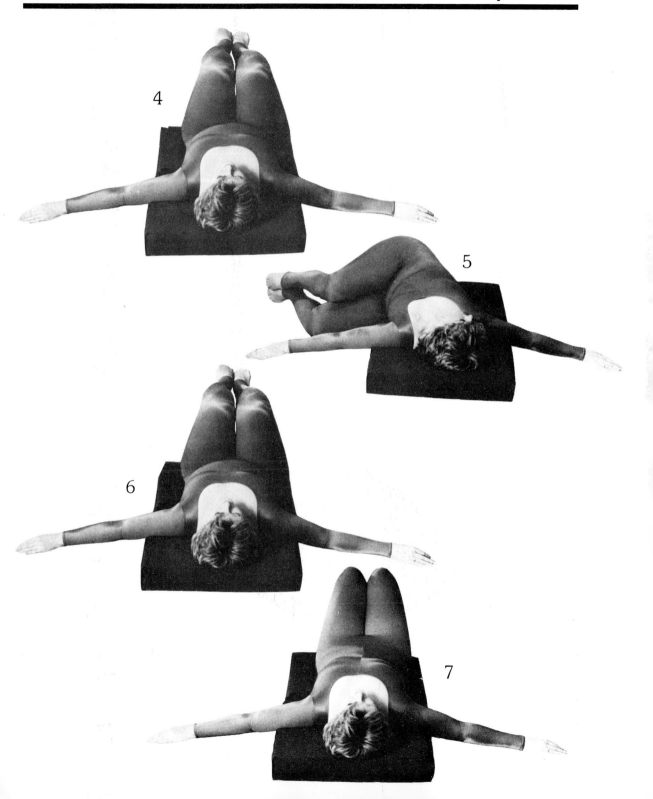

The sitting exercise

This exercise helps improve your sitting position. It also stretches, aligns, and strengthens those torso muscles.

I sit erect with my arms extended overhead. I inhale and exhale comfortably three times. On the third inhale, I bend my torso forward from the pelvic joints. My arms extend forward as I reach my torso out. Then, I roll down one vertebra at a time until my head relaxes on my knees.

I hang there a few seconds with my arms relaxed by my sides. I'm breathing easily. Then I inhale and slowly begin rolling up my spine, while contracting the abdominals into the spine. I finish off by extending my arms overhead, shoulders relaxed and torso as "tall" as possible.

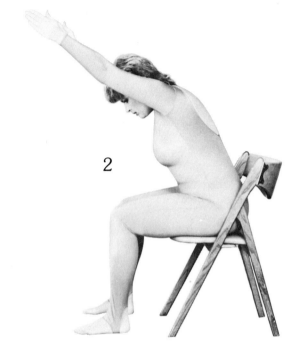

2

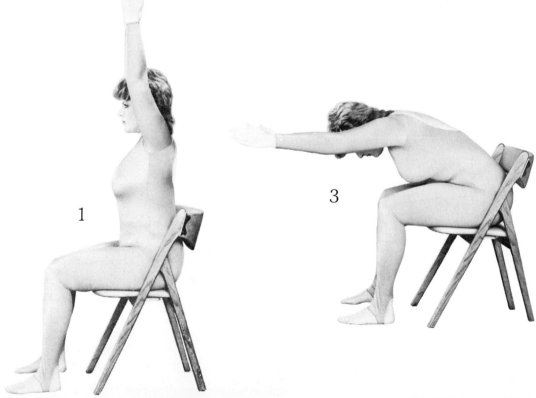

1

3

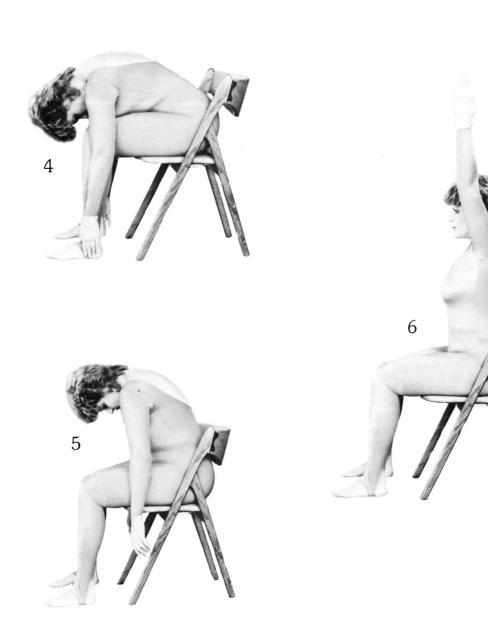

PART FOUR

BEYOND THE NEW YOU: LATER

CHAPTER ELEVEN

WELCOME OVERACHIEVER

You've made it through the whole shape-up program at least once. Well, this chapter is my advanced course for Big Beauties who yearn for more—or is that less? Actually, you'll get a little of both. I'll give you a *more* demanding food plan and a tougher approach to exercising. As a result, there should be a bit *less* of you eventually.

Don't start worrying again about starvation diets or round-the-clock running. These are just some suggestions for taking your efforts to the next level. You'll still have your fantastic new fuller-figure look. But maybe we can make it even more naturally healthy, energy packed, and glamorous.

However, let's first concentrate on keeping the progress we've already made. You don't want to push yourself ahead too quickly. A sudden disappointment might lead to heavy backsliding, rather than miraculous gains. Here's a practical plan that allows you to get comfortable with your recently improved body. Take some time to *really* make it your own.

MAINTAINING THE NEW YOU

Think of *maintenance* as a grace period. It's a manageable, slightly easier interval between more challenging shape-up cycles. This is your chance to level off at a desirable plateau. Believe me, it beats falling back into another valley of despair.

My maintenance program is designed to let

you eat a little more without putting on weight. Of course you won't be *losing* any pounds either. The idea is simply to stabilize both your body size and life-style. You want to develop a routine that can be sustained happily for months or even years.

I strongly suggest that you continue your shape-up exercises during the maintenance. Pep-stepping, biking, or swimming are all pleasant enough activities to fit into a long-term situation. You don't have to escalate them to a more demanding level. Just do them often! They'll cover up minor excesses at the dinner table and keep your body toned.

Let's start off by raising the limit on your calorie intake. Your daily allowance should be somewhere between eighteen hundred and twenty-seven hundred calories. There can't be one convenient number that works for everybody. Each woman's weight balances out at a different point. I'm sure you're all familiar with the variables that have to be taken into consideration. But I'll give you a quick rundown just the same. Try to measure how much each one affects your personal calorie quota.

First, take a good look at *how tall* you are and the size of your bone structure. The bigger you are, the more calories you can consume comfortably. A five-foot-tall woman won't be able to hold her weight down if she matches mouthfuls with somebody my height. My body requires more calories to function properly. Those calories are also more widely dispersed.

Another factor to consider is your *age*. I know a lot of women get better as the years pass. Hey, I'm banking on that myself. But your metabolism does slow down. Women just don't burn up calories as easily once they hit their thirties. Think about all those teenagers who eat up a storm without adding an ounce of fat.

The last variable to ponder is your *degree of activity*. A woman who works at a sedentary job all day should keep her calorie intake down. That's especially true if she comes home every evening just to sit in front of the television. Exercise regularly and your calorie allowance will go up proportionally.

Okay, you now have a fair idea of where your calorie-break-even point winds up. This will help you to prepare psychologically for the kind of food plan you'll be on. There's a lot more leeway in a twenty-seven hundred-calorie day than you'll get in an eighteen hundred-calorie one. Still, we should take the time to narrow down the calorie quota even further.

Begin the maintenance program by adding only three hundred calories to the fifteen hundred calories per day permitted during the shape-up. Stay at eighteen hundred calories daily for a week. At the end of the first week jump on the scale. (It's a necessary evil for a short while.) If there's no noticeable weight gain, then forge on.

For the second week add another three hundred calories daily. Once again weigh in at the end of the week. Holding your own? Add yet another three hundred calories a day for the third week. However, the day you register a pound or two rise in weight, stop. Stop cold! You're overeating, and you must cut back the calories to where you were the week before.

There's more to the maintenance than the extra calories you're allowed to eat. We still have to be concerned about how those calories are consumed. Retain the minimeal method of eating. Also, remember to eat from wisely balanced food groups. In essence, your daily diet should consist of 65 percent carbohydrates (50 percent complex and 15 percent simple sugars), 30 percent protein found in vegetables or meats, and 10 percent fats (5 percent saturated, 5 percent poly- and mono-unsaturated).

By the way, build up your carbohydrates before the fats or proteins. You'll keep your weight at the break-even point with less of a struggle. Master all the maintenance tips, and yo-yoing could be out of your life forever.

THE DIET OF CHAMPIONS

After six to eight weeks of maintaining a certain weight, you should firmly stabilize at that level. From here on you're destined to get better—lighter too. This is a perfect time to switch to "the Diet of Champions." I say it's for champions because everything about it builds winners.

On this tighter food plan you're allowed one thousand calories a day. That's few enough calories to lose more than three pounds per week. Yet, it's still enough calories to fuel a busy, athletically active body. And, as you'll see later, you're going to be playing quite a bit.

In order to maximize the power of those one thousand calories, we're staying with the whole Food Exchange concept. Therefore, optimum nutritional value and balance is guaranteed. A safe, potent vitamin-supplement schedule will also be added. Stick with everything the diet has to offer and you could wind up in the best shape of your life.

Like any change in diet, you should once again check in with your doctor, who, by now, should be absolutely in awe of what you've accomplished. Still, he or she might need an extra dose of assurance about such an ambitious venture. So, tell him you'll be on the one thousand calories for only a week. Then, it's back to maintenance for a week.

The one week on and one week off can be continued until you reach the weight you're hoping for. After the initial week, it's merely a matter of desire. But don't rush to make any commitments you'll regret later. Calm down and assess what's expected of you.

I suggest you take a gander at what *one thousand calories a day* breaks down to in terms of Food Exchange units: Meat Group—4 units; Bread Group—4 units; Milk Group—2 units; Vegetable Group—3 units; Fruit Group—3 units; Fat Group—1 unit. There's no stretching units or going over what's allotted either.

Are you still with me? All right, now let's tackle the vitamin program. Cutting down your food intake often means a loss of certain vitamins or minerals you're used to having. Less calories also leaves you a lot less to burn for energy. Vitamin supplements can more than pick up the slack.

But please don't get carried away! Too much of a particular vitamin can be toxic. On the other hand, a very small quantity of the same vitamin might be relatively useless. You need a strong but safe amount that falls somewhere in the middle. Here's a list that will help you find what you're after. According to the latest data available, these are the maximum daily doses of each vitamin group you can take without fear of toxicity:*

Vitamin A	5,000 I.U.†
Vitamin D	400 I.U.
Vitamin E	100 I.U.
Vitamin C	100-500 mg
Vitamin B_1	5 mg
Vitamin B_2	5 mg
Vitamin B_3	10 mg
Vitamin B_6	10 mg
Vitamin B_{12}	10 micrograms
Pantothenic acid	100 mg
Inositol	100 mg
Choline	100 mg
Folic acid	400 micrograms
Para-aminobenzoic acid (PABA)	50 mg
Calcium	400-800 mg
Magnesium	200-400 mg
Iron	10-14 mg
Chromium	10-40 micrograms
Selenium	50-100 micrograms
Manganese	10-15 mg
Copper	1-3 mg
Zinc	10-20 mg

If you want more information about vitamin supplements, seek out a qualified nutritionist.

*Reproduced from Your Health Under Siege: Using Nutrition to Fight Back, copyright © 1981 by Jeffrey Bland. Reprinted with permission of Stephen Greene Press, Brattleboro, VT.

†International Units

Many chiropractors are quite knowledgeable about vitamin therapy. Or, you can even have a simple blood analysis done. From the results a more exact picture of your vitamin needs can be put together.

SERIOUS FUN-ERCISES

Along with new fitness comes a craving for greater challenges—and results. So I'll give you some general ideas about how to push the exercise throttle a little farther forward. Hopefully, it will do more for your body without sacrificing enjoyment. After all, staying in shape should still be fun rather than work.

By now you'll be displaying more flexibility, strength, and stamina. Your advanced activities will depend on these improvements. Whatever you do, don't rush ahead too quickly. Intensify your exercises slowly, one step at a time. This is not a race to super conditioning.

The Group One sports—biking, pep-step walking, jumping rope, swimming—are done without instructors. The rate of advancement is left strictly to your discretion. Use muscle fatigue and shortness of breath as a measuring stick. When goals or the people around you exceed your limits, drop out. We want to tone bodies, not create martyrs.

For starters, let's make the warm-ups a little more extensive. I recommend adding one or two of the posture exercises on a regular basis. The hip and lower-back relievers are far more effective than bend overs. Sure, the posture exercises are more time consuming. But your back will think they're well worth it. The sitting exercise is a great addition for the bikers. Aligning, stretching, and strengthening torso muscles make it easier to sit properly for hours on end. What's the sense of preparing your legs for pumping if your torso gives out just as you're hitting your stride? And sooner or later all bike riders look to cover long distances.

In fact, distance is the key to revving up your bike routines. Steady fifteen-minute rides one way and then back are highly effective, but they don't leave you much room for growth. Pedaling faster for those fifteen-minute jaunts is all you can do. Yet there's a limit to how fast you can pedal without wrapping yourself around a tree.

I think you should get into bike "touring." These are bike rides of varying distances— two, five, ten or even twenty miles—spread out over an afternoon, day, or weekend. They're done in groups, which should provide companionship and encouragement. Most groups have a mixture of expert, mediocre, and novice bikers. You can stride along with the people who fit your ability.

The pace on these tours is usually moderate but steady. Often the terrain being covered is scenic—country roads, woods, coastal routes, *et cetera*. You'll even find package holidays for bikers at some travel agencies. Primarily, make your choices by the distance to be ridden. Everything else becomes secondary.

Pep-steppers should go along a similar path. Like the bikers, your main avenue for growth is distance. Hiking is the ideal solution. It gives you a chance to expand your walking horizons, while extending your workouts. Hikes of fairly short, medium, and long

distances are available. Write to state or national parks for information about scenic hiking trails. Make sure you take the ruggedness of the terrain into consideration.

Rope jumpers should still be working their way toward that elusive fifteen-minute nonstop. You won't need greater challenges for a long time to come. Swimmers can also keep to the same general aerobic approach they've been following. Just go right on adding distance until you reach about a half mile. Then work at doing that half mile at a faster and faster pace.

Group Two sports are more closely controlled by either an instructor or your ability to compete. Dancers usually have to wait for their teachers' permission to move up to a more advanced class. Sometimes just asking for a more challenging class will let the teacher know that you're ready. You can also request additional routines for the level you're at. Anyhow, nobody ever argued over a little extra practice.

Your tennis and racquetball workouts will automatically intensify as your skills improve. Volleys will be sustained longer, and games should become more demanding. Increased stamina is another plus. You'll have the energy not only to play harder, but longer and more often. Try to get involved in local tournaments. They're usually broken down into beginner, intermediate, and expert ratings. You can pick up some great pointers from fellow competitors.

Both cross-country skiing and snorkeling can be stepped up by joining groups. There are fantastic snorkeling and scuba-diving (the next logical move) vacations for all levels.

Once again, the instruction you get on these extended trips will push you along at a much faster rate. Skiers will learn how to handle steeper hills and tighter areas. Snorkelers and divers will master deeper waters, stronger currents, and longer periods of time in the water.

All the advanced exercising will greatly enhance your sense of confidence and pride.

I hope you've enjoyed every aspect of your quest for glamour. An important part of being a Big Beauty *is* happiness. It shows in your eyes, style of dress, grooming, eating habits, posture, and general health. People see a contented woman in the most favorable light.

When happiness is harder to find, don't hesitate to look deep within yourself. You should be cultivating a positive self-image that transcends temporary moods or situations. Like glamour, everything comes down to an "I won't be denied" attitude. And it works like a charm.

Just look in the mirror for the living proof!

INDEX